THE pilot's COMPLETE
MEDICAL GUIDE

Budds'
Thanks'

THE pilot's complete
MEDICAL GUIDE

by Richard B. Yules, M.D.

Foreword by Lt. Gen. Paul W. Myers, U.S.A.F.
Preface by Robert S. Poole, M.D.

JASON ARONSON, INC. • New York • London

This work was supported by a grant from the Ear, Nose, and Throat Foundation, Incorporated.
Typist: Lynne Monaghan
Proofreader: Rebecca S. Lilien
Artist: Karen Karlsson

Photographs courtesy of Ken Franz.

Library of Congress Cataloging in Publication Data
Yules, Richard B., 1940-
  The pilot's complete medical guide.

  Bibliography: p. 205
  Includes index.
  1. Aviation medicine. 2. Air pilots—Diseases and hygiene. I. Title.
RC1062.Y84   616.9′80213   82-6676
ISBN 0-87668-604-8   AACR2

Manufactured in the United States of America.

To my constant co-pilot,
Lila, and my three favorite
passengers, Branch, Dawn,
and Brooke.

CONTENTS

Foreword

Medical conditions that are potentially hazardous are a critical part of aviation medicine. Aviation Medical Specialists are continuously conducting research and reviewing case histories in order to clearly define acceptable and safe medical limitations.

This volume is a compendium of medical data ranging from Federal Aviation Administration physical examination details to anatomical descriptions of the inner ear. All the information here assists those involved in aviation to understand better the whys and wherefores of physical malfunctions, particularly as they apply to aircraft operation.

The expanding world of aviation involves ever-increasing numbers of people who fly or who are flown. They will gain a deeper understanding of human physiology after reading or referring to this unusual text. It is a ready reference.

Dr. Richard B. Yules' aviation background plus his medical acumen have produced this useful document, which will contribute greatly to aviation safety.

Lt. Gen. Paul W. Myers (Ret.)
Former Surgeon General
United States Air Force

PREFACE

Although this book was written primarily for the civilian pilot, its scope and content make it a valuable reference for the practicing aviation medical examiner as well as others involved with the myriad pilots who ply the skies for commerce, defense, medicine, and just fun.

The author brings more than 20 years of training, experience, and practice to this effort, which covers everything from the physical examination to FAA forms, flight physiology, and anatomical function. It is spiced with enough personal experience to make its perusal more pleasant and instructive.

This book is dedicated to the more than 800,000 active American pilots, as well as to all airmen worldwide. It is hoped that their use of this treatise will make their flying more enjoyable and, more importantly, far safer for themselves and for their passengers.

Robert S. Poole, M.D.
Past President
Civil Aviation Medical Association

INTRODUCTION

Flying touches so many of us. As of January 1980 there were 814,667 active airmen certificates in circulation. Above and beyond the number of actual fliers, the United States aerospace industry had total sales of $37 billion. Excluding commercial flights, to which so many of our fellow travelers have been exposed, over 38 million hours were flown, encompassing 4,619,900,000 passenger miles. We can safely say that flying affects most Americans, if not as fliers, then as passengers and benefactors of the aerospace economy.

With such a marked impact on America, why, then, is no book available relating flying to the airman and passenger? I feel there is such a need. To fill the gap, this book has been written.

The purpose of this book is to describe the FAA physical as it applies to the pilot. But the purpose extends to the passenger as well. It is hoped that pilot and passenger alike will benefit from knowledge of the flying environment and how the environment interrelates with their physical well-being. It is hoped that an understanding of aircraft safety, and the investigations of the accidents that result from a failure to fly safely, will be of interest to all. This book is dedicated to the men and women who shuttle us through the air, who fly to keep our country free, and to those of us who simply sit back, relax, and enjoy the trip.

Acknowledgments

I am indebted to so many people who have made this book possible. My mentor, Dr. Philip Burke, initiated my FAA examiner career and cannot be thanked enough. My partners, Drs. Marshall J. Zamansky and Stephen R. Kurland, have encouraged and supported my efforts, sometimes increasing their work load as a result of my writing this book. My entire office staff at the Haelen Medical Center and at the Ear, Nose, and Throat Foundation, Inc., headed up by Ellie Reidy and our aerospace typist, Lynne Monaghan, have put in extra hours to meet the deadlines of this manuscript.

My physician's assistant and pilot, Bob Palmer, has continually provided the inspiration as well as the basis upon which this book is predicated. My thanks to John J. Cahill, D.O., Regional Flight Surgeon, and to Jon L. Jordan, M.D., Chief of the FAA Aeromedical Standards Division, for proofreading to ensure accuracy with all current regulations. Rebecca S. Lilien's proofreading has also been a great help. Without the efforts of my parents, both of whom worked to support my college and medical school studies, this book never would have been published.

CHAPTER 1

The FAA Physical

The AME

So you need a pilot's medical certificate. The first step—whether for a student pilot or for an already licensed pilot—is to find an AME.

AME stands for Aviation Medical Examiner. Your AME is a representative of the Federal Aviation Administration, is reappointed annually, and is authorized to perform your pilot or flying physical. As of December 1978, there were 7,554 AMEs throughout the USA. Over half of these examiners are pilots themselves, and some 15 percent were formerly military flight surgeons. All have a vital interest in serving your needs as a pilot. AMEs are specifically trained to screen pilot physicals and to examine and advise pilots. They conduct a half-million special examinations each year. In 1978, 565,534 applications were processed. In order to provide you with the best of care, AMEs must attend an FAA three-day update seminar at least every five years—training for which they are not compensated.

AMEs are located throughout the country,

mostly in major cities. Flight instructors and fixed-base operators (FBOs) usually can advise you as to the name of the local AME, and the FAA publishes listings of all AMEs in regional, national, and international publications usually available through airport managers. The Yellow Pages of some areas' telephone directories have a classified section entitled "Aerospace Medicine," which also lists AMEs. Physicals are performed as a service by some 441 Air National Guard and Air Force facilities. Make certain to telephone ahead for approval and an appointment. You may call your local General Aviation District office or the regional flight surgeon listed under U.S. Government, Department of Transportation. If all else fails, write the FAA Aeromedical Certification Branch, P.O. Box 25082, Oklahoma City, Oklahoma 73125.

The AME's Obligation

The overwhelming obligation of your AME is to you and to aviation safety. He or she is responsible for seeing to it that you are physically safe in the cockpit and that you pose no threat to others. The philosophy of medical certification and standards has been well outlined in FAA publications. The levels of concern, of course, extend beyond the individual to society in general. The interest of society must be served by the FAA and consequently by its representative, the AME. This concern exists on three levels: "1. people who pilot aircraft and people who do not; 2. people who are pilots and those who are passengers; 3. those who fly and those on the ground whose person or property may be affected by aircraft operations" (FAA-AM-71-25). Thus, it is evident that the AME has a dual responsibility. He or she is most anxious to keep you in the air and to keep you healthy; he is obligated, further, to see to it that you do not injure yourself or others in your plane, or on the ground. As a result, an AME is required by law to report to the FAA any physical and/or mental defect that might influence your ultimate performance as a pilot. That is not to say that you shouldn't turn to an AME when you do have a problem. He or she is usually the best qualified person to evaluate any problem (physical or emotional) with regard to its effect on your flying. Your AME should be consulted for your own benefit.

Cost

The pilot physical is a thorough evaluation of the major sensory systems, such as eyesight and hearing; in addition, an evaluation of the cardiac, respiratory, and neurological system is made. The fee is not set by the FAA, but by the AME. The current practice is to charge the prevailing rate for a thorough physical exam in the AME's local community, although most pilots report that the AME physical costs slightly less than a physical at their private doctor's office. Fees ranged from about $30 to $50 in 1980. When a Class I examination requires an additional test, such as an electrocardiogram, the extra test is followed by an additional charge. Any specialty consultations that are requested by the FAA and are unobtainable from your AME, will of course be more costly.

Physical Classes

There are three basic classes of FAA medical examinations (see Figure 1-1):

1. First Class: Examination for a first class physical is required every six months and is usually reserved for airline pilots.

Figure 1-1 indicates the minimum class physical requirement for a variety of flying activities. The Class I physical required for an airline transport pilot contains the stiffest requirements and is valid for the shortest period of time. The Class III requirements are more lenient and the physical is valid for a greater period of time.

MINIMUM CLASSES OF MEDICAL CERTIFICATION

REQUIRED FOR AIRMAN ACTIVITY	CERTIFICATE
Airline Transport Pilot	First Class
Air Traffic Control Tower Operator	Second Class
Commercial Lighter-Than-Air Pilot	Second Class
Commercial Pilot	Second Class
Center Controllers	Second Class
Flight Engineer	Second Class
Flight Service Station Controllers	Second Class
Flight Navigator	Second Class
Private Pilot	Third Class
Student Pilot	Third Class
Glider Pilot	None
Student Glider Pilot	None

2. Second Class: Examination for a second class physical is required every 12 months and is usually reserved for commercial airmen flying for hire.
3. Third Class: Examination for a third class physical is required of every private and student pilot and must be performed once every two years.

Only certain AMEs are designated to perform Class I physicals. The designation of these AMEs is noted in the AME Manual by an asterisk preceeding their names. A Class I physical will still serve as a Class II or Class III physical after a six-month interval has expired—a Class I physical is good for one year as a Class II physical and for two years as a Class III physical. Similarly, a Class II physical, when your expiration date has arrived, may be used an additional year as a Class III physical. A Class III physical expires after two years.

Time of expiration is taken from midnight on the last day of the month during which you are certified. Thus, if you were certified on November 10 and had a Class III medical certificate, the certificate would expire at midnight on the last day of November two years from the date of your physical. You can obtain 30 free days in some months by having your physical performed on the first day of the month; thereafter it will not expire for an appropriate period following the last day of the month in which it was issued. Waivers, "statements of demonstrated ability," may generate more frequent examinations, such as every six months.

The vast majority of physicals performed in the U.S. are Class III types. Of the approximately 500,000 medical certificates issued each year, two-thirds are Class III (approximately 20 percent are for new airmen). U.S. citizenship is not required for any physical class, but spoken English is a requirement, as is reading, and applicant comprehension of the English language.

The Student Pilot Certificate

The student pilot medical certificate differs in three ways from a medical certificate issued after you have your pilot's license:

1. The term "Student Pilot Certificate" is added to the front of the medical certificate (see Figure 1-2).
2. The certificate is yellow instead of white.
3. The student pilot medical certificate also contains an area on its reverse side for instructors' endorsements (see Figure 1-3).

Student pilots may take flying lessons with an instructor without having a medical certificate but may not solo until they have one. For this reason, most pilots first arrive at the AME's doorstep after their instructor has indicated to them that they are ready to solo. Once the student pilot has his yellow medical certificate in hand, a signature on the reverse side by a certified

UNITED STATES OF AMERICA
DEPARTMENT OF TRANSPORTATION
FEDERAL AVIATION ADMINISTRATION

AA-3967278

MEDICAL CERTIFICATE_____CLASS
AND STUDENT PILOT CERTIFICATE

THIS CERTIFIES THAT *(Full name and address)*

DATE OF BIRTH	HEIGHT	WEIGHT	HAIR	EYES	SEX

has met the medical standards prescribed in Part 67, Federal Aviation Regulations for this class of Medical Certificate, and the standards prescribed in Part 61 for a Student Pilot Certificate.

LIMITATIONS

STUDENT PILOTS ARE PROHIBITED FROM CARRYING PASSENGERS.

DATE OF EXAMINATION	EXAMINER'S SERIAL NO.

EXAMINER

SIGNATURE

TYPED NAME

AIRMAN'S SIGNATURE

AA FORM 8420-2 (1-67)

Figure 1-2
shows the front of a student pilot certificate. Note that a medical certificate for a student pilot can be obtained in any one of the three classes. The student pilot certificate is so designated on its front and is yellow in color in contradistinction to the regular medical certificate, which is white.

CONDITIONS OF ISSUE: This certificate shall be in the personal possession of the airman at all times while exercising the privileges of his airman certificate. As a medical certificate, it is temporary for a period of 60 days as a student pilot certificate, it is temporary for a period of 90 days. If no notice to the contrary is received within such periods, it will remain in effect until the expiration dates as provided in Sections 61.19 and 61.23 of the Federal Aviation Regulations, unless modified or recalled by proper authority. The holder of this certificate is governed by the provisions of FAR Secs. 61.53, 63.19, and 65.49(d) relating to physical deficiency.

CERTIFICATED INSTRUCTOR'S ENDORSEMENTS FOR STUDENT PILOTS
I certify that the holder of this certificate has met the requirements of the regulations and is competent for the following:

	DATE	MAKE AND MODEL OF AIRCRAFT	INSTRUCTOR'S SIGNATURE	INSTRUCTOR'S CERTIFICATE NO.	EXP. DATE
A TO SOLO THE FOLLOWING AIRCRAFT					
B TO MAKE SOLO CROSS-COUNTRY FLIGHTS		AIRCRAFT CATEGORY			
		AIRPLANE			
		GLIDER			
		ROTOCRAFT			

NOTICE: Any alteration of this certificate is punishable by a fine not exceeding $1,000, or imprisonment not exceeding 3 years, or both

Figure 1-3
shows the back of the student pilot certificate. The student pilot certificate's back differs from the back of a regular medical certificate in that there is room for endorsements of your instructor to convert your medical certificate into a pilot's license.

instructor allows the student to solo. When he has completed all of his pilot requirements, the same medical certificate is signed on the back by the airman's instructor.

After you have earned your pilot's license, the student pilot certificate stands as both your license and medical certificate. Thus, if you had a Class III medical certificate that was issued while you were a *student* pilot, that certificate would be valid as a Class III certificate for two years following the end of the month during which it was issued. It's a good idea to get your flight physical after your first hour or two of pilot training. In this way, if there is a medical problem that may preclude your passing, you can work on it during your training period, correcting the problem so that you will pass the exam.

The Physical—An Overview

There is no cause for concern if this is your first or student pilot FAA physical. The FAA physical is no more difficult than a routine medical examination, which most people have had annually for many years and which has been required for everything from a truck driving license to entry into the Armed Services, to a screening physical prior to a minor surgical procedure. On arrival at your local AME's office, you will be asked to fill out the front sheet of FAA Form 8500-8 (see Figure 1-4). Be sure to fill in all blanks!

After completion of this short history, you will most likely be asked for a urine specimen so that the analysis can be undertaken while the remainder of your physical is in progress. You can then anticipate a hearing test, a vision test, a blood pressure analysis, and then undressing for a complete physical. Once the history, physical, and laboratory studies have been reviewed by the AME, he will indicate whether or not you qualify for the medical certificate. If you do qualify, he

COPY OF FAA FORM 8500-9 (MEDICAL CERTIF- **AA-**
ICATE), OR FAA FORM 8420-2 (MEDICAL/STU-
DENT PILOT CERTIFICATE) ISSUED.

**MEDICAL CERTIFICATE_____CLASS
AND STUDENT PILOT CERTIFICATE**

THIS CERTIFIES THAT *(Full name and address)*

DATE OF BIRTH	HEIGHT	WEIGHT	HAIR	EYES	SEX

has met the medical standards prescribed in Part 67, Federal
Aviation Regulations for this class of Medical Certificate.

LIMITATIONS

DATE OF EXAMINATION	EXAMINER'S SERIAL NO.

EXAMINER SIGNATURE

TYPED NAME

AIRMAN'S SIGNATURE

*WHEN ISSUED AS A MEDICAL-STUDENT PILOT CERTIFICATE,
the holder has met standards prescribed in Part 61, FAR's for such
certificate, and is prohibited from carrying passengers.*

APPLICATION FOR ☐ AIRMAN MEDICAL CERTIFICATE ☐ AIRMAN MEDICAL AND STUDENT PILOT CERTIFICATE

Please print these items

1. FULL NAME *(Last, first, middle)* | PATH CONTROL

2A. ADDRESS *(No. Street, City, State, ZIP No.)* | 2B. SOCIAL SECURITY No.

County:

2C. PLACE OF BIRTH *(Student pilot applicants only)*

3. DATE OF BIRTH *(Mo., day, year)*	4. HEIGHT *(Inches)*	5. WEIGHT *(Pounds)*	6. COLOR OF HAIR	7. COLOR OF EYES	8. SEX

9A. CLASS OF MEDICAL CERTIFICATE APPLIED FOR | 9B. TYPE OF AIRMAN CERTIFICATE(S) HELD

	AIRLINE TRANSPORT	FLIGHT INSTRUCTOR
FIRST	COMMERCIAL	PRIVATE
	ATC SPECIALIST	STUDENT
SECOND	FLIGHT ENGINEER	NONE
THIRD	FLIGHT NAVIGATOR	OTHER

10. OCCUPATION *(If ATC Specialist, specify position and facility)*

11. EXTENDED ACTIVE DUTY MEMBER OF		12. EMPLOYER
a. AIR FORCE	d. COAST GUARD	
b. ARMY	e. NATL. GUARD	13. LENGTH OF TIME IN PRESENT OCCUPATION
c. NAVY/MARINES	f. NONE	
MILITARY SERVICE NO.		14. PRIMARY TYPE OF FLYING
		BUSINESS / PLEASURE

15. CURRENTLY USE ANY MEDICATION *(Including eye drops)*

YES TYPE AND PURPOSE

NO

TOTAL PILOT TIME		18. HAS AN FAA AIRMAN MEDICAL CERTIFICATE EVER BEEN DENIED, SUSPENDED, OR REVOKED	19. HAVE YOU, AS A PILOT, HAD AN AIRCRAFT ACCIDENT WITHIN THE PAST 2 YEARS	20. DATE OF LAST FAA PHYSICAL EXAM *(If none, state so)*
16. TO DATE	17. LAST 6 MOS.			
CIVIL		YES DATE	YES DATE	
MILITARY		NO	NO	

21. MEDICAL HISTORY – HAVE YOU EVER HAD OR HAVE YOU NOW ANY OF THE FOLLOWING: *(For each "yes" checked, describe condition in REMARKS)*

Yes	No	Condition	Yes	No	Condition	Yes	No	Condition	Yes	No	Condition
		a. Frequent or severe headaches			g. Heart trouble			m. Nervous trouble of any sort			s. Medical rejection from or for military service
		b. Dizziness or fainting spells			h. High or low blood pressure			n. Any drug or narcotic habit			t. Rejection for life insurance
		c. Unconsciousness for any reason			i. Stomach trouble			o. Excessive drinking habit			u. Admission to hospital
		d. Eye trouble except glasses			j. Kidney stone or blood in urine			p. Attempted suicide			v. Record of traffic convictions
		e. Hay Fever			k. Sugar or albumin in urine			q. Motion sickness requiring drugs			w. Record of other convictions
		f. Asthma			l. Epilepsy or fits			r. Military medical discharge			x. Other illnesses

REMARKS *(If no changes since last report, so state)*

FOR FAA USE
REVIEW ACTION CODES

22. HAVE YOU EVER BEEN ISSUED A STATEMENT OF DEMONSTRATED ABILITY (WAIVER)
NO
YES *(Give defects and waiver no.)*

PHYSICAL DEFECTS NOTED ON STATEMENT OF DEMONSTRATED ABILITY (WAIVER)

WAIVER SERIAL NO.

23. MEDICAL TREATMENT WITHIN PAST 5 YEARS

DATE	NAME AND ADDRESS OF PHYSICIAN CONSULTED	REASON

– NOTICE –
*Whoever in any matter within the jurisdiction of any
department or agency of the United States knowingly and will
fully falsifies, conceals or covers up by any trick, scheme, or
device a material fact, or who makes any false, fictitious or
fraudulent statements or representations, or makes or uses any
false writing or document knowing the same to contain any
false, fictitious or fraudulent statement or entry, shall be fined
not more than $10,000 or imprisoned not more than 5 years,
or both. (U.S. Code, Title 18, Sec. 1001.)*

24. APPLICANT'S DECLARATION
I hereby certify that all statements and answers provided by me in this examination
form are complete and true to the best of my knowledge, and I agree that they are
to be considered part of the basis for issuance of any FAA certificate to me. I have
also read and understand the Privacy Act statement that accompanies this form.

SIGNATURE OF APPLICANT *(In ink)* | DATE

FAA FORM 8500-8 (10-75)   SUPERSEDES PREVIOUS EDITION   Form Approved. OMB No. 04-R0089

Figure 1-4
is the medical form, which you will be required to fill out during your physical at your AME's office.
The front sheet of this form (8500-8) gives your physician a history of your flight experience and past
medical conditions. This form is required at each and every physical that you subsequently take.

will issue the certificate right then and there. If federal regulations do not allow the AME to issue you a certificate, the AME will issue you a letter of denial (see Figure 1-29 on p. 30). You are expected to pay for your physical at the time you are seen by the physician.

The physical usually does not take longer than one hour. And it is a good idea for all people to have a similar physical even if they are not applying for a pilot's license. FAR Part 67, "Medical Standards and Certification," is reproduced in Appendix 1 and details the official policy.

Medical History

Your examination by the AME is preceded by your filling out a brief history. Filling out this form alerts the physician to the class of medical certificate for which you are applying. This is important since requirements are more stringent for Class I than they are for Class II physicals and similarly more stringent for Class II than for Class III physicals. The form also provides information that gives the physician a feeling of how active you have been during your flying career and whether or not you have ever required a medical standards waiver (a "statement of demonstrated ability") in the past. The history form also provides specific information that may be important about your past medical problems, and finally, parts of the history provide information that automatically would keep the AME from issuing you a medical certificate, without giving an exam.

It is imperative that the material you present on your medical application be accurate and thorough. You are responsible for providing the AME with any relevant information that might affect your medical status. Read the notice on your application. Part 67 of the FARs deals with medical standards and certification. Section 67.20

makes it clear that if you do not fill out your medical application accurately, there is cause for revoking both your medical certificate and your rating. The specifics should be clearly understood by all airmen:

67.20 Applications, Certificates, Logbooks, Reports, and Records: Falsification, Reproduction, or Alteration.

a. No person may make or cause to be made:

1. Any fraudulent or intentionally false statement on any application for a medical certificate under this Part

2. Any fraudulent or intentionally false entry in any logbook, record, or report that is required to be kept, made, or used, to show compliance with any requirement for any medical certificate under this Part

3. Any reproduction, for fraudulent purpose, of any medical certificate under this Part

4. Any alteration of any medical certificate under this Part.

b. The commission by any person of an act prohibited under paragraph (a) of this section is a basis for suspending or revoking any airman, ground instructor, or medical certificate or rating held by that person.

You have a legal obligation to provide accurate, complete information on your history form. Both you and your AME accept a legal responsibility for assuring that the information provided on your history and physical form is as accurate as possible.

Failure by you to provide accurate information places you in violation of Federal Criminal Law Title 18 USC 1001:

Whoever in any matter in the jurisdiction of any department or agency of the United States knowingly, and willfully falsifies, conceals or covers up by any trick, scheme or device a material fact, or who makes any false, fictitious, or fraudulent statements or representations, or makes or uses any false writing or document knowing the same to contain any false, fictitious, or fraudulent statement or entry, shall be fined not more than $10,000 or imprisoned not more than five years, or both.

The above does not even take into consideration any subrogation that an insurance company might subsequently present against you. Falsifications may make you responsible for losses incurred by your insurance company.

Doubters should read the September 1979 issue of *AOPA Pilot* magazine. A 26-year-old airman was indicted on two counts by a federal grand jury because he represented to the FAA that he had no record of any traffic or other convictions. The U.S. District Attorney, a federal prosecutor, is prosecuting the pilot. The FAA has lifted the airman's medical and commercial pilot's certificate. He faces a 10-year imprisonment and/or a $20,000 fine.

The Medical Examination

The medical examination is an extensive evaluation by the physician (See Figure 1-5, numbers 25–60). Numbers 25–48 comprise the general physical examination conducted by your physician with instruments designed to look into your ears, eyes, nose, and throat; to listen to your heart and lungs and abdomen; and to feel or palpate the various parts of your body to detect pathology, frequently accompanied by a rectal examination. As you can see from numbers 49–55, there is a great deal of emphasis on the examination of the sensory systems, in particular those of hearing and vision.

The qualifications for hearing and eyesight are different in each class of physical and are delineated in Figures 1-6 and 1-7. These figures serve

REPORT OF MEDICAL EXAMINATION

NOR-MAL	CHECK EACH ITEM IN APPROPRIATE COLUMN (Enter NE if not evaluated)	AB-NOR-MAL	NOTES: Describe every abnormality in detail, enter applicable item number before each comment. Use additional sheets if necessary and attach to this form.
	25. Head, face, neck and scalp		
	26. Nose		
	27. Sinuses		
	28. Mouth and throat		
	29. Ears, general (Internal and external canals) (Auditory acuity under item 49)		
	30. Drums (Perforation)		
	31. Eyes, general (Visual acuity under items 50 & 51)		
	32. Ophthalmoscopic		
	33. Pupils (Equality and reaction)		
	34. Ocular motility (Associated parallel movement, nystagmus)		
	35. Lungs and chest (Including breasts)		
	36. Heart (Thrust, size, rhythm, sounds)		
	37. Vascular system		
	38. Abdomen and viscera (Including hernia)		
	39. Anus and rectum (Hemorrhoids, fistula, prostate)		
	40. Endocrine system		
	41. G–U system		
	42. Upper and lower extremities (Strength, range of motion)		
	43. Spine, other musculoskeletal		
	44. Identifying body marks, scars, tattoos		
	45. Skin and lymphatics		
	46. Neurologic (Tendon reflexes, equilibrium, senses, coordination, etc.)		
	47. Psychiatric (Specify any personality deviation)		
	48. General systemic		FOR FAA USE - PATHOLOGY CODE NOS.

49. HEARING		RIGHT EAR				LEFT EAR				50. DISTANT VISION (Standard test types only)			51. NEAR VISION (Use linear values)	
WHISPERED VOICE (STANDING SIDEWAYS DISTANT EAR CLOSED)		FT.				FT.				RIGHT EYE	20/	CORRECTED TO 20/	20/	CORRECTED TO 20/
AUDIOMETER (Decibel Loss)	500	1000	2000	4000	500	1000	2000	4000		LEFT EYE	20/	CORRECTED TO 20/	20/	CORRECTED TO 20/
										BOTH EYES	20/	CORRECTED TO 20/	20/	CORRECTED TO 20/

52. INTRAOCULAR TENSION (Tonometry required for Air Traffic Control Specialist)			53. COLOR VISION (Test used, number of plates missed)
TACTILE	RIGHT EYE	LEFT EYE	
TONOMETRIC			

54. FIELD OF VISION		55. HETEROPHORIA DIOPTERS (Not required for Class Three)				
RIGHT EYE	LEFT EYE	DISTANCE	ESOPHORIA	EXOPHORIA	RIGHT H.	LEFT H.

56. BLOOD PRESSURE			57. PULSE (Wrist)		
RECUMBENT, MM MERCURY	SYSTOLIC	DIASTOLIC	RESTING	AFTER EXERCISE	2 MINUTES AFTER EXERCISE

58. URINALYSIS		59. ECG (Date)	60. OTHER TESTS
ALBUMIN	SUGAR		

61. COMMENTS ON HISTORY AND FINDINGS; RECOMMENDATIONS (Attach all consultation reports, ECGs, X-rays, etc. to this report before mailing)	FOR FAA USE
	CODED
	PUNCHED
	VERIFIED

62. APPLICANT'S NAME	63. DISQUALIFYING DEFECTS (List by item no.)	EXAMINER CODES
HAS BEEN ISSUED ☐ MED. CERTIF. ☐ MED. AND STUDENT PILOT CERTIF. NO CERTIF. ISSUED - FURTHER EVALUATION REQUIRED HAS BEEN DENIED - LETTER OF DENIAL ISSUED (Copy attached)		CLERICAL REJECT

64. MEDICAL EXAMINER'S DECLARATION   *I hereby certify that I personally examined the applicant named on this medical examination report, and that this report with any attachment embodies my findings completely and correctly.*

DATE OF EXAMINATION	AVIATION MEDICAL EXAMINER'S NAME AND ADDRESS (Type or print)	AVIATION MEDICAL EXAMINER'S SIGNATURE

Figure 1-5
is the back of Form 8500-8, which you fill out during your FAA medical examination. This portion of the form is completed by your AME before a copy is sent to the FAA certification office in Oklahoma. You, of course, are not required to (and you should not) fill out any portion of numbers 25 through 64. You should be aware, however, of the type of information that is being evaluated.

MAXIMUM HEARING LOSS (db)

CLASS	(Hz)	500	1,000	2,000
I either ear		25	25	25
II either ear		25	25	25
III better ear		25	25	25
III poorer ear		40	40	40

Figure 1-6
specifies the maximum hearing loss allowable for the different classes of physicals. "Hz" means hertz or cycles per second. Only the three frequencies critical to speech intelligibility are employed in determining disqualifying criteria. If your hearing does not meet the above requirements, a statement of demonstrated ability, a waiver, may be obtained. The AME, however, is required to issue a letter of denial, or forward your application to Oklahoma City for further evaluation.

VISION REQUIREMENTS

CLASS	DISTANT		NEAR	
	UNCORRECTED	CORRECTED	UNCORRECTED	CORRECTED
I and II	20/100	20/20	Any	20/40
III	20/50	20/30	Any	20/60

Figure 1-7
lists the vision requirements for Class I, II, and III physicals. Requirements are different for distant and near vision. Distant and near vision are evaluated separately during your physical. It is possible to have a limitation typed onto your medical certificate that applies only to distant *or* near vision; it is also possible to have a limitation typed onto your certificate that applies to both distant *and* near vision. If your vision does not correct to the required level for the class physical you are obtaining, the AME is not permitted to issue you a medical certificate. It is possible, however, to obtain a waiver with demonstrated flight ability using denial channels.

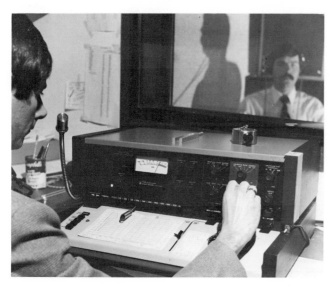

Figure 1-8
illustrates conventional audiometry performed in a sound-attenuated room with an instrument designed to evaluate your hearing at a variety of frequencies. The product of such testing is exhibited in Figure 1-9.

Figure 1-9 demonstrates a conventional audiogram or hearing test performed as part of your FAA physical. The symbols are readily understood if you remember that an open circle refers to the right ear and an "x" to the left ear. An arrow refers to how you hear with a bone conductor in contradistinction to the circle and "x," which demonstrate how you hear with an earphone. Of course, the earphone and bone conductor graphs should superimpose if your hearing is normal. Speech reception threshold is your response to bisyllabic words such as "hotdog," "football," "playground," and the like. Discrimination refers to your ability to comprehend single syllable words that are similar-sounding, such as "wear," "bear," "there," "are," "air." It is this discrimination that diminishes as we get older and this discrimination that decreases especially in noise-induced hearing loss.

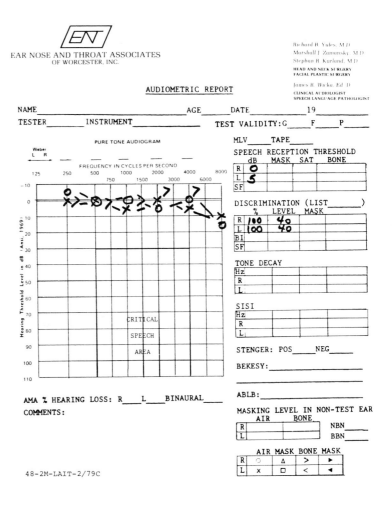

only to summarize the barest essentials of the evaluation. Feel free to ask your AME to read the specific requirements on hearing and eyesight, which are very detailed and specific. They are listed in Appendix 1.

Hearing evaluation can legally be conducted with the whispered voice. Should a problem be detected in hearing, an audiometric or hearing-test evaluation is indicated. This is usually accomplished with a conventional audiometer in a sound-attenuated room (see Figures 1-8 and 1-9).

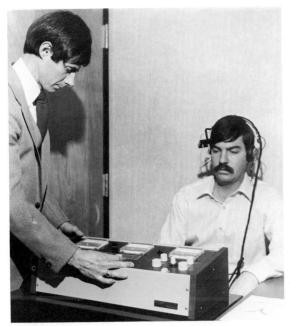

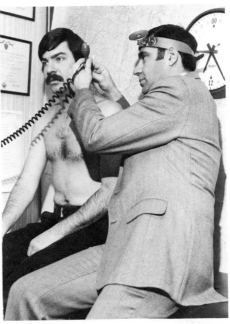

Figure 1-10
demonstrates a tympanometer. A tympanometer does not depend upon your response for an evaluation. Sound and pressure are automatically recorded to demonstrate the resistance and compliance of your middle-ear structures. This results in an excellent evaluation of eustachian-tube function. The product of the tympanometer test, a tympanogram, is exhibited in Figure 1-11.

Figure 1-11
illustrates an otoscopic examination of the ears. The rubber ball of the otoscope provides pressure to determine both patency and mobility of the eardrum. Ability to clear your ears can be determined from mobility of the eardrum when you swallow. Should you have an ear block, the eardrum will not move when air is pushed against it.

It is sometimes also necessary to obtain a tympanogram, which measures compliance and resistance of the eardrum as well as eustachian tube function (see Figures 1-10, 1-11 and 1-12). Should you have any doubts about your hearing capability, request an audiogram; should you have trouble clearing your ears on descent, request a tympanogram.

Visual evaluation is carried out most frequently with a vision tester (see Figures 1-13, 1-14, 1-15, and 1-16). On certain occasions, an ophthalmological or eye-physical consultation may be re-

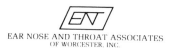

EAR NOSE AND THROAT ASSOCIATES
OF WORCESTER, INC.

Richard B. Yules, M.D.
Marshall I. Zamansky, M.D.
Stephen R. Karland, M.D.
HEAD AND NECK SURGERY
FACIAL PLASTIC SURGERY
OTOLOGY

James R. Wocku, Ed.D.
CLINICAL AUDIOLOGIST
SPEECH LANGUAGE PATHOLOGIST

I M P E D A N C E   M E A S U R E M E N T   R E P O R T   F O R M

NAME _____ AGE_____ DATE _____ 19____
EAR SX. _____ TESTER _____
Test Instrument: Madsen Electro- Acoustic Impedance Bridge, Model Z073

Figure 1-12

shows a tympanogram or impedance - measurement report. We perform these as part of our routine examination, although they are not required by the FAA, and doctors who aren't otologists may not have this equipment available. This allows us to determine whether or not you have good eustachian-tube function and/or whether or not the resistance of your eardrum is normal. This is an excellent measure of whether or not fluid is present behind the eardrum and how you may be expected to perform in rapid descents in terms of ear equilibrium.

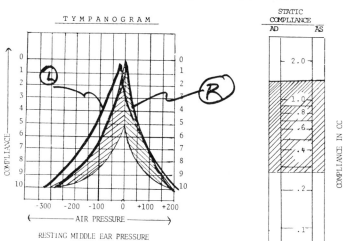

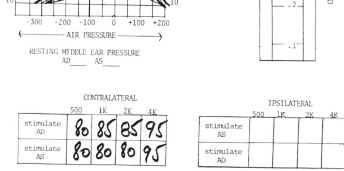

	CONTRALATERAL			
	500	1K	2K	4K
stimulate AD	80	85	85	95
stimulate AS	80	80	80	95

	IPSILATERAL			
	500	1K	2K	4K
stimulate AS				
stimulate AD				

STAPEDIUS REFLEX (HTL)

4 2M LAIT 2/79C   REMARKS _____

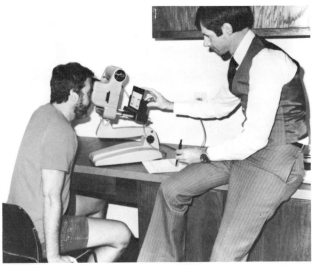

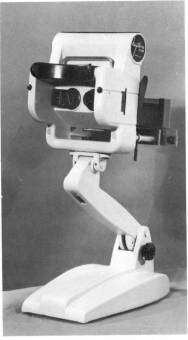

Figure 1-13
illustrates a typical arrangement for evaluation of your vision. Most FAA medical examiners now employ a similar type of vision tester for performing the entire vision screening procedure for every class of physical.

Figure 1-14
shows a typical vision tester frequently used during flight physicals. Near vision, distant vision, eye drift and ability to center the eyes, and color vision are all tested. (Photo courtesy of the Keystone View Company, Davenport, Iowa)

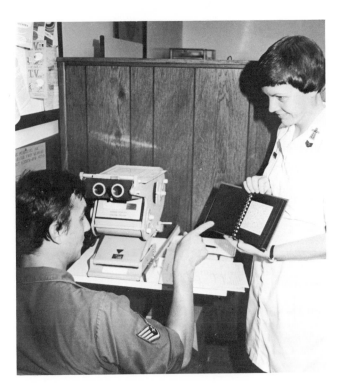

Figure 1-15.
Color vision testing can be accomplished either with a series of plates printed in a book, as noted in this figure, or with a special pattern projected on a Keystone Viewer, as noted in Figure 1-14.

17

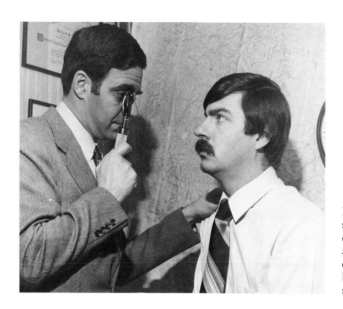

Figure 1-16
shows an AME evaluating a pilot's eyes with an ophthalmoscope. Examination with an ophthalmoscope detects not only ocular problems, but can detect systemic diseases, such as arteriosclerosis or diabetes.

quired. In this case, a form similar to that in Figure 1-17 must be filled out by your eye physician.

Glasses

Wearing glasses and/or contact lenses is not in itself a contraindication to being issued a medical certificate. Your local AME will type this limitation onto your certificate. However, your eyesight must be no worse than the limits listed in Figure 1-7, and your glasses and/or contact lenses must correct your vision properly to the level stated.

A limitation on your license, depending upon

Figure 1-17
is a typical ophthalmological or eye consultation form required under certain conditions for you to obtain a "waiver" or statement of demonstrated ability. Your AME will advise you when such consultation is required. Should you have a known eye deficiency, you would be well advised to bring along a letter from your ophthalmologist prior to your FAA physical. This will save time and expedite obtaining your medical certification. (See pp. 19–20.)

Form Approved : Budget Bureau No. 004-R0163

DEPARTMENT OF TRANSPORTATION - FEDERAL AVIATION ADMINISTRATION	1. DATE
REPORT OF EYE EVALUATION	

2A. NAME OF AIRMAN	2B. DATE OF BIRTH	2C. SEX

3. ADDRESS OF AIRMAN

4. HISTORY—Record pertinent history, past and present, concerning general health and visual problems.

5. HETEROPHORIA—Record phorias, in prism diopters, with and without best lens correction in place *(Use Maddox Rod).*

A. WITHOUT CORRECTION	(1) AT 20 FEET			(2) AT 18 INCHES		
	EXO.	ESO.	HYPER.	EXO.	ESO.	HYPER.

B. WITH CORRECTION *(If any)*	(1) AT 20 FEET			(2) AT 18 INCHES		
	EXO.	ESO.	HYPER.	EXO.	ESO.	HYPER.

6. FUSION—Estimate fusion ability and state methods used in examination. *(Red lens, etc.)*

7. PUPILS—Statement of relative size and reaction of the pupils to accomodation and light, direct and consensual.

8. VISUAL FIELDS—Record results and type of test performed *(Attach field charts, if used)*

9. OPHTHALMOSCOPIC—Describe any variations from normal in either eye on funduscopic examination.

10. SLIT LAMP—Record results of slit lamp examination of each eye where indicated.

11. INTRAOCULAR PRESSURE—Record results and method used.

A. METHOD USED	O.D.	O.S.

12. VISUAL ACUITY *(Snellen linear values)*

A. NEAR VISION	TEST METHOD	UNCORRECTED			LENSES USED	CORRECTED VISUAL ACUITY		
		OD	OS	OU		OD	OS	OU
					CONTACT LENSES ONLY			
					GLASSES ONLY			
					GLASSES WITH CONTACTS			

NOTE - If contact lenses are used, corrected near visual acuity should be determined while these lenses are worn. Indicate if the contact lenses used (if any) were bifocal:

B. DISTANT VISION	TEST METHOD	UNCORRECTED			LENSES USED	CORRECTED VISUAL ACUITY		
		OD	OS	OU		OD	OS	OU
					CONTACT LENSES			
					GLASSES			

NOTE - If contact lenses are used, record after four to six hours wear and then with glasses immediately after removal of contacts. If visual acuity is not the same as for contact lenses, indicate length of time *(within reason)* before vision returns to best obtainable with glasses.

C. KERATOMETER READINGS	IF CONTACT LENSES ARE WORN		BEFORE CONTACT LENSES WERE FITTED *(If available)*	
	O.D.	O.S.	O.D.	O.S.

FAA Form 8500-7 (2-76) SUPERSEDES PREVIOUS EDITION

13. PRESENT PRESCRIPTION (Sphere, cylinder, axis)			
A. CONTACT LENSES		B. GLASSES	
OD	OS	OD	OS

IF CONTACT LENSES ARE NOT USED, OMIT ITEMS 14-19.

14. DATE OF FITTING OF PRESENT CONTACT LENSES (NOTE - Adaptive period of 3 months required)

15. DESCRIPTION OF CONTACT LENSES UTILIZED

A. MANUFACTURER

B. TYPE OF LENSES (Corneal, scleral, lenticular, single-cut, bifocal, toric, non-rotating, special shape, etc.)

C. COLOR AND GRADE OF TINTING, IF ANY, AND REASON FOR TINTING (Cosmetic, light, sensitivity, etc.)

16. BACKUP SET—Is a backup set of spectacles available for immediate use?

17. EXAMINATION FREQUENCY—Indicate frequency of periodic followup examination.

18. SYMPTOMS OR ABNORMAL CONDITIONS—Note any lacrimation, photophobia, loss of lens, or evidence of corneal injury or edema, etc., requiring treatment and/or interruption of contact lens wearing. State results of slit lamp or biomicroscopic examination of cornea.

19. TOLERANCE (Periods of Wear)

A. DAYS CONTACT LENSES WORN DURING LAST MONTH	B. DAILY WEARING TIME IN HOURS

20. PROFESSIONAL EVALUATION—Indicate your professional opinion and any other comment or additional observations.

21A. TYPED NAME AND ADDRESS OF EYE SPECIALIST	21B. SIGNATURE OF EYE SPECIALIST

☆ U.S. GOVERNMENT PRINTING OFFICE: 1976-211-372/655

Figure 1-17 (continued)

UNITED STATES OF AMERICA
DEPARTMENT OF TRANSPORTATION
FEDERAL AVIATION ADMINISTRATION

MEDICAL CERTIFICATE_____CLASS

THIS CERTIFIES THAT *(Full name and address)*					
DATE OF BIRTH	HEIGHT	WEIGHT	HAIR	EYES	SEX

has met the medical standards prescribed in Part 67, Federal Aviation Regulations for this class of Medical Certificate

LIMITATIONS

Holder shall wear glasses that correct for distant vision & possess glasses that correct for near vision while exercising the privileges of an Airman Certificate.

DATE OF EXAMINATION	EXAMINER'S SERIAL NO
EXAMINER SIGNATURE	
EXAMINER TYPED NAME	
AIRMAN'S SIGNATURE	

FAA FORM 8500.9 10-73 SUPERSEDES PREVIOUS EDITION

Figure 1-18
demonstrates a typical limitation for vision that may be issued by your AME during your physical. Ordinarily, the "limitation" portion of your medical certificate will say "none." Should you have an eye deficiency that can be adequately corrected by glasses, the AME will type in a limitation similar to the one noted.

UNITED STATES OF AMERICA
DEPARTMENT OF TRANSPORTATION
FEDERAL AVIATION ADMINISTRATION

MEDICAL CERTIFICATE_____CLASS

THIS CERTIFIES THAT *(Full name and address)*					
DATE OF BIRTH	HEIGHT	WEIGHT	HAIR	EYES	SEX

has met the medical standards prescribed in Part 67, Federal Aviation Regulations for this class of Medical Certificate.

LIMITATIONS

Not valid for night flight or by color signal control.

DATE OF EXAMINATION	EXAMINER'S SERIAL NO.
EXAMINER SIGNATURE	
EXAMINER TYPED NAME	
AIRMAN'S SIGNATURE	

FAA FORM 8500-9 (1-67)   SUPERSEDES FAA FORM 1004-1

Figure 1-19
is an example of a medical certificate issued to a pilot with deficient color vision. Because of his poor color vision, the pilot is restricted to day flight and is not allowed to use tower color control signals for communication.

your individual situation, will result in a statement on your license as in Figures 1-18 and 1-19.

The only laboratory study required of a pilot to obtain medical certification is a urinalysis. No blood studies are required except under special circumstances, which might be indicated by your history and/or subsequently requested by the FAA. The urinalysis can be performed on a small specimen, delivered to the AME in a clean specimen cup. The test is readily performed by using

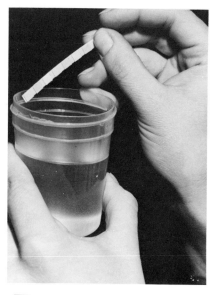

small filter paper reagent strips (see Figures 1-20 and 1-21).

Don't be thrown by the semantics of medicine. Sometimes you just have to say, "Say again." I had a patient very early in my practice who arrived for his flight physical. "Charlie," I said, "Micturate in that specimen container." "What's that, doc?" said Charlie. I said, "Charlie, urinate in that specimen container." "Don't understand,

Figure 1-20
demonstrates the reagent strips that are employed in performing a urinalysis for the FAA physical. By simply placing a dipstick with numerous chemicals embedded upon it into your urine, many determinations can be made. (Courtesy Ames Company)

A URINE PROFILE OF DIFFERENTIAL DISEASE FINDINGS

	RENAL	HEPATIC	PANCREATIC	GASTROINTESTINAL
ph	Renal tubular acidosis Bacterial infections Chronic renal failure		Diabetic acidosis	Diarrhea Pyloric obstruction Vomiting Malabsorption
Protein	Nephrotic syndrome Pyelonephritis Glomerulonephritis Kimmelstiel-Wilson syndrome Malignant hypertension			
Glucose	Lowered renal threshold Renal tubular disease		Pancreatitis Diabetis mellitus	Alimentary glycosuria
Ketones		von Gierke's disease (glycogen storage disease)	Diabetic acidosis	Vomiting Diarrhea
Bilirubin		Complete and partial obstructive jaundice Viral and drug-induced hepatitis Cirrhosis	Carcinoma of the head of the pancreas	Choledocholithiasis
Blood	Hematuria in Acute nephritis Passive congestion of the kidneys Calculi Malignant papilloma Renal carcinoma Nephrotic syndrome Polycystic kidneys	Hematuria in: Cirrhosis (impaired prothrombin function)	Hemoglobinuria in: Kimmelstiel-Wilson syndrome	Hematuria in: Diverticulosis of the colon
Nitrite	Significant Bacteriuria			
Urobilinogen		Obstruction of the bile duct Liver cell damage Cirrhosis	Carcinoma of the head of the pancreas	Suppression of the gut flora (antibiotic therapy)

doc." "But Charlie, urinate in that container over there." "Doc, I still don't read you." "Charlie, damn it, piss in that cup." "From here, doc?"

HEART EXAMINATION

The cardiac, or heart, examination is accomplished by listening to the heart with a stethoscope, feeling the strength and equality of the peripheral pulses, and looking for any congestion of veins, which might indicate cardiac difficulties. (See Figures 1-22, 1-23 and 1-24.) Unless there is a history of cardiac difficulties, a Class II or III examination requires nothing more sophisticated

CARDIOVASCULAR	OTHER	
Congestive heart failure	Dehydration Starvation Low-carbohydrate diets	Acetazolamide therapy Metabolic acidosis Metabolic alkalosis Emphysema
Benign hypertension Congestive heart failure Subacute bacterial endocarditis	Toxemia of pregnancy Gout Brown-spider bite Acute febrile state	Carbon tetrachloride poisoning Electric-current injury Potassium depletion Orthostatic proteinuria
Coronary thrombosis	Pheochromocytoma Hyperthyroidism Acromegaly	Shock Pain Excitement
	Starvation Low-carbohydrate diets Eclampsia Hyperthyroidism	Trauma Chloroform or ether anesthesia

Congestive heart failure in the
  presence of jaundice
	Recurrent idiopathic jaundice of
	  pregnancy
		Noxious fumes
		Chloropromazine hepatitis

Hematuria in:
Bacterial endocarditis
Hemoglobinuria in:
Intravascular hemolysis
Hypertension with renal
  involvement
	Hematuria in:
	Chronic infections
	Chronic phenacetin ingestion
	Sulfonamide therapy
	Sickle-cell disease
	Hemoglobinuria in:
	Severe burns
		Hemolytic anemias
		Transfusion reaction
		Sudden cold
		Eclampsia
		Allergic reactions
		Multiple myeloma
		Alkaloids—poisonous
		  mushrooms

Congestive heart failure Extravascular hemolysis	Noxious fumes Hepatitis associated with infectious mononucleosis Thalassemia	Pernicious anemia Hemolytic anemias Chlorpromazine hepatitis

Figure 1-21 demonstrates the urine profile of differential disease findings. Note the incredible number of conditions that can be detected from a simple urinalysis during your FAA physical.

in the way of cardiac evaluation. A Class I examination, however, requires an electrocardiogram (EKG) or heart tracing on the applicant's first examination following his 35th birthday and annually in Class I applicants age 40 and over. The EKG examination (see Figure 1-25), consists of an electrical tracing of microvolt electrical impulses generated by the heart and picked up by a series of electrodes on the skin overlying your chest. The tracing is subsequently transferred to a heat-sensitive paper and submitted to the FAA for analysis. A sample electrocardiogram is shown in Figures 1-26 (p. 27) and 1-27 (p. 28). Should the electrocardiogram be abnormal, a cardiac evaluation may be required, and you will be notified by the FAA. Should the tracing be flat, forget about flying.

Figure 1-22.
An important part of your physical is auscultation or a stethoscopic evaluation of your heart. The examiner is noting the regularity of the rhythm and the presence of any unusual sounds, which could signal imminent heart problems.

Figure 1-23.
One requirement that is part of the flight physical (#57) is to check the pulse rate after exercising. Here a physician's assistant monitors the pilot's pulse two minutes after exercise.

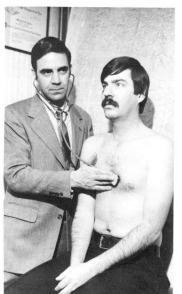

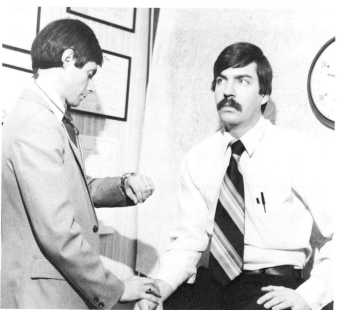

BLOOD PRESSURE LIMITS (mm/Hg)

	CLASS I	CLASS II & III
Age	Maximum	
20–29	140/88	170/100
30–39	145/92	
40–49	155/96	
50	160/98	

Class I, II, III—continuous medication not allowed.

Figure 1-24 illustrates the limits on blood pressure imposed on the different classes of physicals. Class I requirements are the most stringent. Class II and III requirements are lenient enough that the vast majority of Americans —regardless of age—will comply with the requirements. Note that all readings are without the effects of medication. Taking continuous medication for blood pressure control is disqualifying, although it is possible to obtain a waiver.

If your history indicates a myocardial infarction (heart attack), congenital heart disease, or certain cardiac diseases, or your physical indicates that you have a cardiac problem, then the AME is required to issue you a letter of denial, (see Figure 1-28 on p. 29), or to send the entire examination to Oklahoma City for further evaluation. If a cardiac consultation has been obtained, and an appropriate electrocardiogram and chest X-ray submitted to the FAA Administrator, it is possible that your flying will not be terminated.

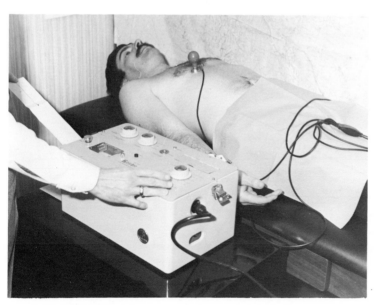

Figure 1-25 demonstrates how an electrocardiogram is taken and shows leads attached to the pilot's extremities. The electrocardiogram is perfectly safe. Microvolt pick-up from the electrical activity of the heart muscle is amplified many times and results in the printed tracing shown in Figure 1-26. This photograph of an electrocardiograph technician illustrates the suction cup—placed on the patient's chest—that is responsible for picking up the V1–6 leads noted in Figure 1-27.

CLINICAL RECORD	ELECTROCARDIOGRAPHIC RECORD	PREVIOUS ECG ☐ YES ☐ NO

CLINICAL IMPRESSION	MEDICATION	☐ EMERGENCY ☐ BEDSIDE ☐ ROUTINE ☐ AMBULANT

AGE	SEX	RACE	HEIGHT	WEIGHT	B. P.	SIGNATURE OF WARD PHYSICIAN	DATE

RHYTHM	AXIS DEVIATION (QRS)	RATES
		AURIC. VENT.

INTERVALS	P WAVES
PR QRS QT	

QRS COMPLEXES

RS—T SEGMENT	T WAVES

UNIPOLAR EXTREMITY LEADS (*Specify*)

PRECORDIAL LEADS (*Specify*)

SUMMARY, SERIAL CHANGES, AND IMPLICATIONS:

(*Continue on reverse*)

NO. ECG	SIGNATURE OF PHYSICIAN	PATIENT'S IDENTI-FICATION NO.	DATE

PATIENT'S IDENTIFICATION (*For typed or written entries give: Name—last, first, middle; grade; date; hospital or medical facility*)	REGISTER NO.	WARD NO.

ELECTROCARDIOGRAPHIC RECORD
(Attach Tracings to SF—507)

Standard Form 520
Revised April 1968
General Services Administration &
Interagency Comm. on Medical Records
FPMR 101—11—809—3
520—105
GPO 1972 O - 461 - 631

Figure 1-26.

26

Figure 1-26.
Follow me through an explanation of the electrocardiographic record, reading from left to right and from top to bottom. The previous EKG, or electrocardiogram, should be checked "yes" or "no." If a previous electrocardiogram has been performed, this provides a means of comparison, should an abnormality be detected. Thus the examiner can determine if a condition is new, old or progressing. The clinical impression is the overview of the entire reading, and in pilots will almost always read "within normal limits (WNL)." Medication taken is important since cardiac, antihypertensive, and endocrine medications will frequently affect the electrocardiogram. For a normal FAA physical, the AME will have checked "routine."

The age and sex are important since they determine the normal limits of an electrocardiogram. So do height, weight, and blood pressure. Finally, every electrocardiogram should be dated. An electrocardiogram must be taken within 90 days before an exam but not necessarily on the day of a Class I physical examination. Rhythm is important since any irregularity is an abnormality and must be investigated further. Ordinarily, this block will read "NSR" or normal sinus rhythm, which indicates that the electrical pacemaker or sinus of the heart is functioning properly. The axis deviation is determined by reading Roman numeral I and Roman numeral III (seen in Figure 1-27).

A vector analysis allows the examiner to determine whether the left or right side of the heart is enlarged, thus indicating early pathology. The rates of both the auricle and ventricle should, of course, be identical, and in most of us nonrunners they fall in the 70-beats-per-minute range. The intervals of **PR**, **QRS**, and **QT** are measurements of the different segments of the heartbeat. The **PR** interval is the distance between the auricle beat and the ventricle beat and is usually 0.12 seconds. The **QRS** interval is the time during which the electrical activity flows over the ventricle, or main portion of the heart, and is usually 0.04 seconds. The **QT** interval is the time it takes for the ventricle to repolarize and get ready for the next beat, and is usually 0.40 seconds.

Similarly, P waves, **QRS** complexes, **RS** segments and T waves all refer to analysis of normal heights of the segment in question. These heights are a function of age and heart rate. Unipolar extremity leads **R–F** refer to the electrical activity picked up from foot and arm electrodes. The primary function of these leads is to detect abnormalities in axis deviation of the heart. The precordial leads refer to V1–6, noted in Figure 1-27, and are taken by the suction cup pickup, shown in the cardiogram photograph of Figure 1-25. Abnormalities not detectable on Roman numerals I-III and letters **R–F** can sometimes be picked up from the anterior chest leads.

Any serial change from previous electrocardiograms would be noted and the presumed clinical diagnosis would then be indicated. Thus, with a very careful vector and rhythm analysis, an electrocardiogram is a complex reading that can indicate many different diseases of the cardiovascular system.

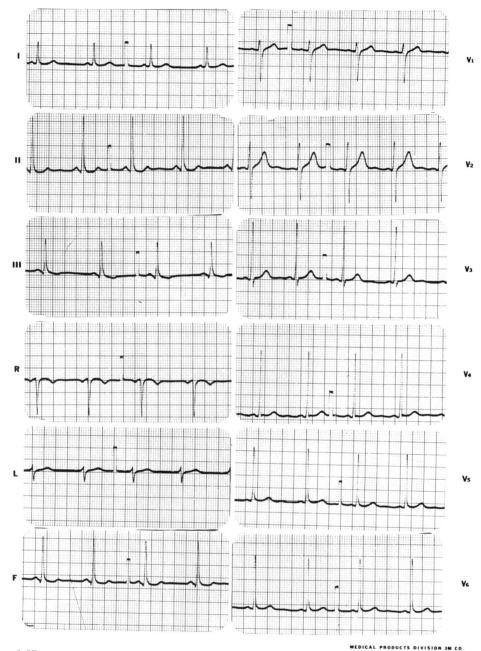

I

II

III

R

L

F

V₁

V₂

V₃

V₄

V₅

V₆

MEDICAL PRODUCTS DIVISION 3M CO.

Figure 1-27
is a typical mounted electrocardiogram. The designation on the side of the tracings refers to different leads, which pick up different electrical axes of heart activity (see Figure 1-26). By evaluating the different leads, your physician is able to determine a host of cardiac difficulties—frequently before an acute problem has occurred. Should you have had a myocardial infarct or a heart attack, the electrocardiogram will usually demonstrate this.

28

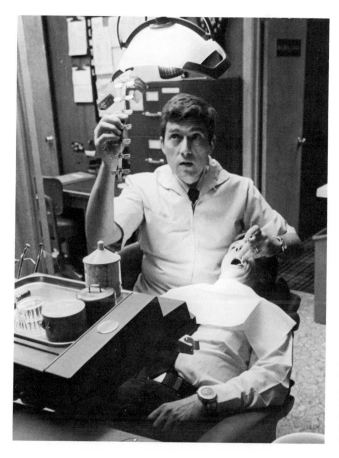

Figure 1-28
shows a periodic dental examination. Early detection and treatment
of dental-oral conditions can prevent sudden pain while flying,
which can impair or even incapaci-
tate the flier's split-second judgment. Air trapped in the teeth,
gums, or bone can expand by the
same mechanism as can air in the
sinus cavity or middle-ear space.
Although a dental examination is
not specifically required for medical
certification, a wise pilot will maintain an optimum level of oral health
at all times.

REAsoNs foR MEdicAl DisquAlificATioN

Your local AME is required to deny you a
medical certificate if you omit or refuse to sign
Item 1-24 in the medical history, which states that
all answers are correct. He must also disqualify
you if you have ever been denied medical certification, unless you hold a statement of demonstrated ability covering the cause for denial. There
are nine disorders for which a medical history or
clinical diagnosis generates a mandatory denial:

DEPARTMENT OF TRANSPORTATION
FEDERAL AVIATION ADMINISTRATION

Consideration of your application for airman medical certificate
and the medical examination given you on   ,
discloses that you do not meet the standards prescribed in
section(s)
of the Federal Aviation Regulations because of the following
conditions:

Therefore, pursuant to the authority delegated to me by the
Administrator of the Federal Aviation Administration, your application
for issuance of an airman medical certificate is hereby denied.

This denial does not constitute an action of the Administrator
under section 602 of the Federal Aviation Act and is subject to
reconsideration by the Federal Air Surgeon or his authorized
representative. A request for such reconsideration may be made
pursuant to section 67.27, Part 67 of the Federal Aviation
Regulations, by submitting a written request in duplicate to the
Federal Air Surgeon, ATTN: Chief, Aeromedical Certification Branch,
P.O. Box 25082, Oklahoma City, Oklahoma 73125. In the event no
application for reconsideration is made within thirty days of this
action, you will be deemed to have acquiesced in the denial and to
have withdrawn your application for a medical certificate.

You are advised that it is unlawful under the Federal Aviation
Regulations for you to exercise airman privileges unless you hold
an appropriate medical certificate. Further, it is unlawful for
the holder of a medical certificate to exercise such privileges
if he has a known medical history or condition which makes him
unable to meet the physical requirements for that certificate.

_____
Aviation Medical Examiner

Figure 1-29
is a typical letter of denial (**FAA Form 8500-2**). Causes for denial are discussed in the text, as are methods for appealing or overcoming the denial.

_____
Designation Number

FAA Form 8500-2 (1-67)   FAA AC 73-911

1. A character or behavior disorder leading to overt acts
2. A psychotic disorder
3. Chronic alcoholism
4. Drug addiction
5. Epilepsy
6. Disturbances of consciousness without cause
7. Myocardial infarction (heart attack)
8. Angina pectoris (heart pain)
9. Diabetes requiring medication for control

Neither the regional flight surgeon, the chief of the aero-medical certification section, nor the Federal Air Surgeon can issue a ticket for any of the above nine denial reasons. Each case must pass through the exemption procedure by way of the Administrator.

Any airman undergoing continuous treatment with a variety of medications, including barbiturates, tranquilizers, steroids, and/or antihypertensive or antihistamine medication must also be denied his medical certificate. A full 6 percent of applications require further action prior to approval, but only 1.5 percent of all applications are medically disqualified.

Recourse to Medical Certificate Denial

If your medical certificate is denied by the AME, he will issue you a letter of denial similar to Form Letter 8500-2 illustrated in Figure 1-29. A copy of the form letter will be given to you and forwarded to the Aeromedical Certification Branch of the Federal Aviation Administration along with the FAA copy of your physical 8500-8. If you are denied a medical certificate, you have one of three courses of action:

1. Accept the denial. This rejection will not jeopardize your right to submit a future application.
2. Request, within 30 days, further consideration by the Federal Air Surgeon.
3. Petition for exemption from the published standards if you have a mandatory denial condition (see Figure 1-30).

Reconsideration by the Federal Air Surgeon

If you wish to appeal the AME's decision of denial to the Federal Air Surgeon, the appeal

ROLE OF THE AVIATION MEDICAL EXAMINER
IN FAA MEDICAL CERTIFICATION

THE AME:

Represents the Administrator in the performance of delegated functions (acts as FAA official).

Examines applicants to obtain information essential to determining their qualifications for medical certification (obtains facts).

Decides whether applicants meet the pertinent medical standards prescribed in Federal Aviation Regulations, Part 67 (makes discretionary decision)

Issues or *Denies* airman medical certificates (initiates FAA action).

FAA Administrative Proceedings

1. Review of AME's action on medical certificate.
2. Cases of approval: no further action.
3. Cases of non-approval: certificate issued may be recalled; certificate denied may be issued.
4. Who besides AMEs may issue medical certificates:
   a. Regional Flight Surgeon (after review & evaluation)
   b. Aeromedical Certification Branch (after review & evaluation)
   c. Federal Air Surgeon (after evaluation or upon orders of NTSB)
   d. Administrator (upon grant of an exemption)
5. Actions resulting from AME's certification of unqualified airmen:
   a. Action by Regional Flight Surgeon to effect surrender of medical certificate.
   b. In cases where procedure 5a is ineffective, FAA Regional Counsel issues Emergency Order of Revocation.
   c. Decision by National Transportation Safety Board required if revocation is appealed by airman.

Actions Open to the Airman

Appeal of denial to:

1. Regional Flight Surgeon
2. Aeromedical Certification Branch
3. Federal Air Surgeon
4. FAA Administrator (Exemption cases)
5. National Transportation Safety Board Examiner
6. Full National Transportation Safety Board
7. U. S. Court of Appeals

Figure 1-30
shows denial and review procedures for medical certification (continued on pp 33-34).

DENIAL AND REVIEW PROCEDURES   (Section 602)

(within 60 days after initial action by AME)

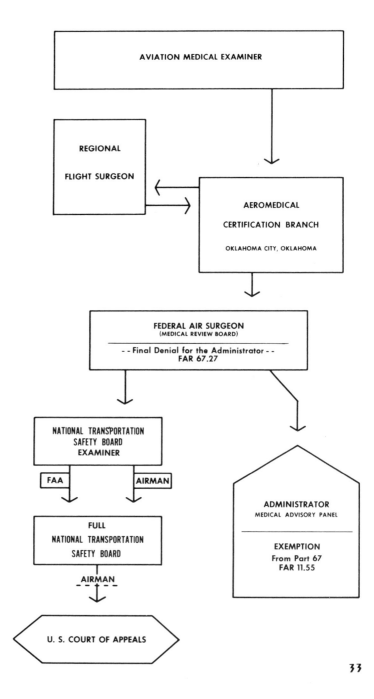

EXAMINATION
Evaluates the history
Evaluates the physical
Acts in accordance with Part 67

REVIEW-EVALUATION
Obtains necessary clinical records,
   test reports, etc.
Evaluates medical problem cases,
   concurs, or reverses

REVIEW-EVALUATION
Evaluates cases, concurs, or reverses
Supplies Regional Flight Surgeon with
   problem case clinical records, etc.
Recommends action to Federal Air
   Surgeon

RECONSIDERATION
Review by Federal Air Surgeon
Investigates medical history
Requests special medical tests
Evaluates for limited issuance
Obtains legal advice, etc.
Concurs in, modifies, or reverses
   previous action taken.

HEARING
Medical witnesses
Record evidence
Legal arguments
Initial decision

APPELLATE REVIEW
Reviews evidence, record, briefs, etc.
Issues Order

JUDICIAL REVIEW

C   FAA AC 70-4653

Figure 1-30 (continued).

AVIATION MEDICAL EXAMINER

REGIONAL

FLIGHT SURGEON

AEROMEDICAL

CERTIFICATION BRANCH

OKLAHOMA CITY, OKLAHOMA

FEDERAL AIR SURGEON
(MEDICAL REVIEW BOARD)

- - Final Denial for the Administrator - -
FAR 67.27

NATIONAL TRANSPORTATION
SAFETY BOARD
EXAMINER

FAA   AIRMAN

FULL
NATIONAL TRANSPORTATION
SAFETY BOARD

AIRMAN

ADMINISTRATOR
MEDICAL ADVISORY PANEL

EXEMPTION
From Part 67
FAR 11.55

U. S. COURT OF APPEALS

33

REVOCATION AND APPEAL PROCEDURES (Section 609)

(Required when 60 days elapse before further action is taken)

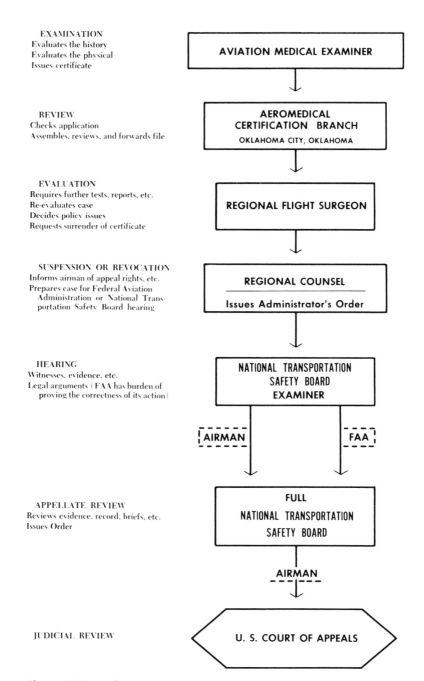

EXAMINATION
Evaluates the history
Evaluates the physical
Issues certificate

AVIATION MEDICAL EXAMINER

REVIEW
Checks application
Assembles, reviews, and forwards file

AEROMEDICAL CERTIFICATION BRANCH
OKLAHOMA CITY, OKLAHOMA

EVALUATION
Requires further tests, reports, etc.
Re-evaluates case
Decides policy issues
Requests surrender of certificate

REGIONAL FLIGHT SURGEON

SUSPENSION OR REVOCATION
Informs airman of appeal rights, etc.
Prepares case for Federal Aviation Administration or National Transportation Safety Board hearing

REGIONAL COUNSEL
Issues Administrator's Order

HEARING
Witnesses, evidence, etc.
Legal arguments (FAA has burden of proving the correctness of its action)

NATIONAL TRANSPORTATION SAFETY BOARD EXAMINER

AIRMAN   FAA

APPELLATE REVIEW
Reviews evidence, record, briefs, etc.
Issues Order

FULL NATIONAL TRANSPORTATION SAFETY BOARD

AIRMAN

JUDICIAL REVIEW

U. S. COURT OF APPEALS

Figure 1-30 (continued).

procedure is outlined in the letter of denial shown in Figure 1-29. Remember that your request for reconsideration should be instituted within 30 days of your denial. The Federal Aviation Act of 1958 is the basis for your reconsideration, which is carried out in an informal manner by the Federal Air Surgeon or his designee. You can submit any and all data that you think might support your case. You may be asked to undergo a medical flight test to determine whether you have a physical limitation that may impair your ability to operate an aircraft safely.

Should your reconsideration request be approved, you will be issued a Statement of Demonstrated Ability (FAA Form 8500-15), which is then typed onto your physical (see Figure 1-31).

UNITED STATES OF AMERICA
DEPARTMENT OF TRANSPORTATION
FEDERAL AVIATION ADMINISTRATION

STATEMENT OF DEMONSTRATED ABILITY

This form cannot be used in lieu of a medical certificate; it should be attached to your medical certificate.

AIRMAN'S NAME AND ADDRESS

CLASS OF MEDICAL CERTIFICATE AUTHORIZED   WAIVER SERIAL NO.

LIMITATIONS

PHYSICAL DEFECTS

BASIS OF ISSUANCE

☐ OPERATIONAL EXPERIENCE ☐ SPECIAL PRACTICAL TEST ☐ SPECIAL FLIGHT TEST

☐

FOR THE FEDERAL AIR SURGEON

DATE

SIGNATURE (TO BE SIGNED IN INK)

NAME AND TITLE (TO BE TYPED)

FAA FORM 8500—15 (12-69) FORMERLY FAA FORM 779

Figure 1-31
is an illustration of a Statement of Demonstrated Ability (SODA) issued by the Federal Air Surgeon through his aeromedical certification branch. Most SODAs are based on demonstrated ability. On occasion, medical consultation will provide the information necessary for issuing a waiver.

Waivers and Exemptions

Should you not comply with requirements for medical certification—be it by history or physical examination—you should not despair. The mechanism is clearly established to effect a waiver or exemption should this be required in your individual case. Let's look at some examples of situations that have resulted in exemption for the pilot.

Many items in the history are automatically disqualifying and require that the AME deny your medical certificate. For example, if you are taking thyroid medication, your AME cannot issue you a certificate; but he can enclose a recommendation along with a summary of your medical history to the regional flight surgeon, who may then issue you your medical certificate. You may fly in spite of the fact that you are currently on medication providing that you do not have to change your medication levels and that you remain asymptomatic. It's that simple.

So don't try to hide any medical history, but understand that the FAA and its representatives (the AMEs) are under legal obligation to follow certain courses of action. In the long run, however, if you are really capable of flying medically, you can usually be assured of receiving your certificate in an expeditious, minimally aggravating manner.

Now let's take the extreme case of a double amputee. Arthur Zervas is a flight instructor in spite of the fact that he has no legs. This action required demonstrated ability with a representative from the General Aviation District Office (GADO). Nonetheless, even under circumstances where many men would have despaired, the pilot was able to pursue an avocation that others might have thought impossible.

In March of 1980, history was made when, for the first time, a pilot who had undergone coronary artery bypass surgery was returned to flight status. The airline pilot, 51-year-old Captain James D. Schwartz, of Frontier Airlines, underwent coronary bypass surgery five years prior to his return to flight status. Although he was denied by the FAA, the five-man National Transportation Safety Board approved his return to flight status. He was due to begin training to take command of a Boeing 737 twin-jet airliner. Thus, the appeal process for even extreme cases may provide a mechanism by which you may be returned to flying status.

Reconsideration (waiver) procedures can extend not only to severe motor disabilities but also to severe sensory disabilities. For example, a totally deaf person may obtain a pilot's license and be certified medically, but with certain restrictions. A deaf person would not be allowed to enter any zone of a controlled (radio) airfield. He would, however, be able to land on an uncontrolled airport even if Unicom were there, since there is, of course, no requirement to use Unicom. The message is clear: If a person really desires to fly, even though he/she has a disability, a mechanism for reconsideration is available. Airmen can take heart from the fact that in 1979, of 683 reconsideration decisions rendered by the Federal Air Surgeon, about one-third (248) resulted in issuance of airmen medical certificates, while two-thirds (435) were denied. For those fortunate enough to be granted waivers and for the others as well, the government did not simply turn its own deaf ears to their problems.

Nor are the sympathies of the medical profession confined to civilian pilots. There is a recent success story of an Air Force pilot who was thought crippled for life. He recently logged 1,000 hours in an F-15:

"In July of 1968, Lt. Col. Thomas C. Skanchy parachuted out of an F-4 Phantom jet while taking off from Seymour Johnson Air Force Base, in North Carolina. His chute failed to deploy, and he was nearly killed. He suffered two fractured legs, a broken ankle, broken pelvis, broken back, and multiple head and internal injuries. His back-seater did not survive. We are told in *Air Force* magazine (February 1980) that his doctors thought he would never walk again, let alone fly. After four months in traction, Colonel Skanchy was discharged from the hospital wearing a total body cast. But Colonel Skanchy had the will to survive and the perseverance to exercise in spite of his cast and crutches. Following assurance by neurosurgeons that there was no permanent brain injury, and after appropriate rehabilitative therapy, Colonel Skanchy was cleared to fly again. A former patient, Colonel Skanchy, now 40 years of age, commands a fighter weapon squadron where he instructs aerial combat and ground delivery tactics in our most modern Air Force tactical fighter, the F-15. So, in spite of severe injuries, be it a civilian or military person, the will and ability to fly can put you back in the driver's seat. Don't give up hope, and don't stop trying."

The *classic* example of the successful amputee is beautifully set down in Paul Brickhill's *Reach for the Sky*. This is the story of a pilot who lost both legs while learning to fly, only to regain a flying position and become one of Britain's leading aces. The true story of Douglas Bader demonstrates the will of the pilot in challenging medical review boards in order to get back into the seat of a fighter. Finally, as a double amputee, following a series of appeals, Doug Bader found himself in a Spitfire above the English Channel. He became a leading ace with over 30 downed planes to his credit. He bailed out over France, at which point his artificial limbs became entangled in his plane, and he came near to destruction, but he survived.

Final Appeal of Medical Denial

Should reconsideration by the Federal Air Surgeon and/or an attempt to be exempt from the regulations fail, you still have the right to petition the National Transportation Safety Board within 60 days of your denial. Although all procedures up to this point are informal and do not require a hearing, petition to the National Transportation Safety Board is a legal move to ascertain if the Federal Aviation Regulations have been applied fairly. The Board appoints a hearing examiner who conducts the hearing under strict legal procedure in a geographic area close to you. It is surely advised that you be represented by an attorney. If your hearing examiner supports your medical certification denial, you still have the option of requesting a review by the full panel of the National Transportation Safety Board. Certainly this sequence of options and appeals has maximized your right, as an airman, to obtain certification, if at all reasonable.

Replacing a Lost Medical Certificate

Lost or defaced medical certificates may be replaced by sending $2 to the Oklahoma City Aeromedical Certification Branch, P.O. Box 25082, Oklahoma City, Oklahoma 73125. Your request should include the following pieces of information:

1. Your name and date of birth
2. Your address and Social Security number
3. Class of medical certification
4. Place and date of examination
5. Name of examiner
6. What happened to the original certificate

The medical branch receives 80,000 letters and/or telegrams per year. Some 35,000 telephone requests are answered annually, and 2,500,000 medical files are maintained. Over 2,200 applications for medical certification are received daily. So, have a little patience. Remember that over 250,000 applications (47 percent of input cases) are rejected by the computer and require manual adjudication by professional personnel. In the midst of this, they will still get your lost medical certificate back to you.

Responsibility

The ultimate responsibility for safe flying is yours. The ultimate responsibility for maintaining and insuring that your physical condition is adequate for safe flying is yours.

FAR 61.53 states most emphatically concerning "Operations during physical deficiency" that "no person may act as a pilot in command, or in any other capacity, as a required pilot flight crew member while he has a known physical deficiency that would make him unable to meet the physical requirements for his current medical certificate."

Enough said. If you think that you might have a condition that limits your flying ability, you are required not to fly. You should have your condition evaluated by an Aviation Medical Examiner.

The life you save may be yours, or it may be the life of another.

CHAPTER 2

Illness and the Pilot's Environment

The Pilot's Environment

The pilot's environment is a constantly changing portion of atmosphere. Almost all flying takes place in the troposphere (see Figures 2-1 and 2-2), the division of our inner atmosphere that contains weather, has variable temperatures, contains water vapor and turbulence, and extends up to approximately 33,000 feet. It is the pressure of this atmosphere that accounts for some of the problems encountered by the flier, such as hypoxia, dysbarism (decompression sickness), and frostbite. The atmosphere invokes a third dimension by taking our feet off the ground, and that accounts for sensory illusions and motion sickness. The pilot's environment is important to understand because the effects of the environment have such profound consequences on how we function physically.

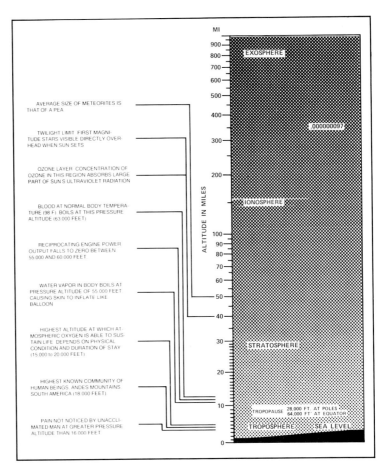

Figure 2-1
demonstrates the different levels of the atmosphere extending from the troposphere through the exosphere. Our flying takes place in the troposphere.

The Atmosphere

The composition of the atmosphere is remarkably constant until about 70,000 feet. It is composed primarily of two gases: nitrogen (78%) and oxygen (21%). The percentage and the pressure of oxygen are especially critical to us; it is the side effect of nitrogen that can be so devastating. The temperature in the troposphere, where almost all flying takes place, decreases approximately 3.5° F per 1,000 feet of ascent. Thus temperatures at a variety of altitudes can be anticipated as follows:

DIVISION AND COMPOSITION OF THE ATMOSPHERE

ATMOSPHERIC STRATA AND THEIR ALTITUDE RANGE

		Spheres	Layers	Approximate Ht.
Atmosphere		Outer	Exosphere		5000 km
					700 km
	Inner	Ionosphere	F layers	140 – 200 km
			E layer	85 – 140 km
			D layer	80 – 85 km
		Stratosphere	Upper mixing layer	50 – 80 km
			Warm layer	30 – 50 km
			Isothermal layer	11 – 30 km
		Troposphere	Tropopause	8 – 11 km
			Advection layer	2 – 8 km
			Ground layer	2m – 2 km
			Bottom layer	0 – 2 m

Troposphere—division containing most weather; characterized by variable temperatures, presence of water vapor and turbulence
Tropopause—transition zone between troposphere and stratosphere
Stratosphere—characterized by lack of water vapor, no weather (except tops of thunderstorms)—in lowest layer (isothermal layer) temperature is constant – 55°C
Ionosphere—zone of ionized air produced by short ultraviolet radiation

IMPORTANT MEDICAL AND FLIGHT OPERATIONAL LEVELS WITHIN THE ATMOSPHERE

Beginning of subcritical hypoxia	At 4km (13,123 ft)
Critical hypoxia	At 8 km (23,000 ft)
Boiling of body fluids, or ebullism (Armstrong Line)	At 20 km (65,000 ft)
The limit for aerodynamic navigation (von Karman Line)	From 60 – 80 km (37 – 49 mi)
The official demarcation line between atmosphere and space	100 km (328,000 ft) (62 mi)
Border of the mechanically effective atmosphere	150 – 200 km (93 – 124 mi)

Figure 2-2 is a breakdown of the division and composition of the atmosphere with relevant medical and flight operational levels within this atmosphere.

Altitude	Temperature
Sea level	50° F
5,000 ft.	41° F
10,000 ft.	23° F
15,000 ft.	5° F
20,000 ft.	-12° F
25,000 ft.	-30° F
30,000 ft.	-48° F
35,000 ft.	-67° F

Up beyond 35,000 feet, the temperature remains remarkably constant. There, pressure decreases with ascent even more rapidly than does temperature. A rule of thumb is to advance the decimal point to the left one digit for every 50,000 feet of ascent. Thus sea level pressure of 760 millimeters mercury (Hg), can be converted as follows:

Sea Level	760 mm Hg
53,000 ft.	76 mm Hg
106,000 ft.	7 mm Hg

An easy way to remember pressure differentials is to remember that at 18,000 feet, the pressure is one-half atmosphere and at 35,000 the pressure is one-quarter atmosphere (179 millimeters mercury). There is a colony of human beings who exist at 18,000 feet in the Andes. But these folks have undergone extreme climatic habituation, which includes increased red-blood-cell mass and the ability of the tissues to subsist at a low oxygen level. To you, 18,000 feet represents 30 minutes of useful consciousness and then unconsciousness.

Hypoxia

So you say you have a small single-engine plane, whose service ceiling is 11,000 feet. You can't suffer from hypoxia, right? Wrong! It is imperative that you realize that you can suffer from hypoxia, even at a relatively low altitude. Hypoxia is easily understood by dividing the

Figure 2-3.
Standardization of terms used in respiratory physiology. In order for you to grasp much of what is published in oxygen instruction booklets, this figure is included so that you might better understand the anatomic or physiologic terms employed in describing respiratory physiology. The tidal volume at any level of activity is really the factor used in determining basic oxygen requirements. In diseased states or when pushed hard, the other reserve volumes can come into play and can markedly affect the duration of your oxygen supplies.

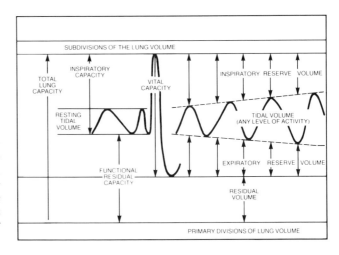

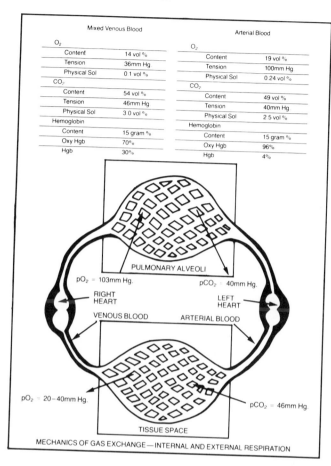

Mixed Venous Blood			Arterial Blood	
O_2			O_2	
Content	14 vol %		Content	19 vol %
Tension	36mm Hg		Tension	100mm Hg
Physical Sol	0.1 vol %		Physical Sol	0.24 vol %
CO_2			CO_2	
Content	54 vol %		Content	49 vol %
Tension	46mm Hg		Tension	40mm Hg
Physical Sol	3.0 vol %		Physical Sol	2.5 vol %
Hemoglobin			Hemoglobin	
Content	15 gram %		Content	15 gram %
Oxy Hgb	70%		Oxy Hgb	96%
Hgb	30%		Hgb	4%

PULMONARY ALVEOLI

$pO_2 = 103$mm Hg. $pCO_2 = 40$mm Hg.

RIGHT HEART   LEFT HEART

VENOUS BLOOD   ARTERIAL BLOOD

$pO_2 = 20-40$mm Hg. $pCO_2 = 46$mm Hg.

TISSUE SPACE

MECHANICS OF GAS EXCHANGE—INTERNAL AND EXTERNAL RESPIRATION

Figure 2-4.
The mechanics of the gas exchange in both internal (tissue space) and external (pulmonary alveoli) respiration. Notice that the pressure of oxygen in the alveoli, which are the exchange portions of the lungs, accounts for the positive pressure, which pushes oxygen into the blood to be carried by the hemoglobin and thence diffused into the cells of the body tissues. It is when the pressure in the pulmonary alveoli drops to the point where there is no positive gradient into the blood and tissues that we become hypoxic and oxygen-starved.

word into two portions: the prefix, *hyp*, means low, and the remainder of the word, *oxia*, means oxygen. Hypoxia is low or inadequate oxygen in the pilot's tissues. In order for you to understand hypoxia, you must have some appreciation of its types, causes, symptoms, treatment, and prevention. (See Figures 2-3 and 2-4.)

Hypoxia can affect anyone at any time, at altitude or at sea level. As a rule of thumb, younger and healthier individuals are less prone to hypoxia than are older or sickly individuals. Nonsmokers and nondrinkers are less prone to hypoxia than are smokers and drinkers.

The single best preparation you can obtain in dealing with hypoxia is to spend a day on an FAA chamber ride at a local Air Force facility. As noted in Figure 2-26 (p. 72), all the background for understanding hypoxia and demonstrating its symptoms and treatment is made available to you in a decompression (or recompression) chamber provided by the Air Force for civilian pilot training. Call your local GADO (General Aviation District Office) and find out the nearest facility at which you can sign up.

The physiological training program of the FAA is available for a $5 administrative fee. If you cannot obtain the information from local sources, write Department of Transportation, Federal Aviation Administration Aeronautical Center, Civil Aeromedical Institute, Physiological Operations and Training Section AAC-143, P.O. Box 25082, Oklahoma City, Oklahoma 73125.

When you have completed this course, you will understand how even below 11,000 feet hypoxia can strike.

Symptoms

It is critical that you be able to recognize your own symptoms of hypoxia. *The most dangerous part of hypoxia is its insidious nature, which makes it difficult to detect.* Detection is further complicated by the euphoria that accompanies hypoxia, which camouflages the upcoming catastrophe. Symptoms vary from person to person, which is why the FAA chamber ride in an Air Force facility is so useful to you; you will learn to recognize your own symptoms. Most people know the classic symptoms of hypoxia, such as headache, fatigue, and irritability; you may have felt them as a hangover but not recognized them as a form of histotoxic hypoxia. At altitude, symptoms such as air hunger, restlessness, dizziness, headache, euphoria, and tunnel vision are more difficult to detect. It is imperative that you learn your own symptoms. Cyanosis or blue lips and fingernails can go unnoticed. Mental and motor degradation, which follow the previously listed symptoms, may occur after it is too late for you to recognize the hypoxia.

Types and Causes

There are four types of hypoxia: 1. hypoxic hypoxia; 2. hypemic hypoxia; 3. stagnant hypoxia; and 4. histotoxic hypoxia. Let's take a look at the cause and the treatment of each type of hypoxia.

Hypoxic Hypoxia is the form of hypoxia that is caused by reduction of oxygen (O_2) in inspired air. As previously mentioned, the pressure envelope surrounding the earth decreases as we ascend. At sea level, there is a total of 760 millimeters mercury of pressure, of which approximately 100 millimeters is oxygen. Since the pressure of oxygen in the blood is only 40, this provides a positive gradient of 60 (100 minus 40) from the lungs to the blood at sea level. If we take our turbocharged Bonanza to 18,000 feet, roughly one-half of sea level pressure is now present, or 380 millimeters of mercury. Somewhere between sea level and 18,000 feet is the point at which the pressure of oxygen in the lungs is inadequate to push all the needed O_2 into the blood. This pressure mark is present at 11,500 feet. So, the requirement of mandating oxygen for use above 12,000 feet is not unreasonable (see Figures 2-5 and 2-6). In fact, as we will discuss in talking about vision and other sensory perceptions, you are far better off using as a rule of thumb, "10,000 feet and over needs oxygen." This will allow you

Figure 2-5.
Remember that prediction of oxygen consumption is only an approximation. When we are working harder, when it is hotter, when we are more excited —under all these circumstances—we invariably use more oxygen.

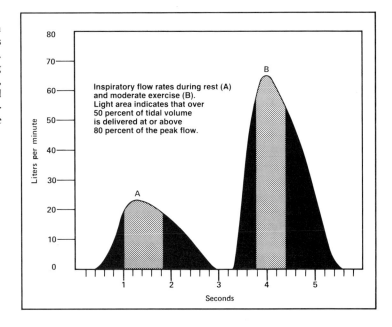

Inspiratory flow rates during rest (A) and moderate exercise (B). Light area indicates that over 50 percent of tidal volume is delivered at or above 80 percent of the peak flow.

a margin of error that corrects for density altitude. The FAA Aviation Medical Series #4 says it all in the title: "The higher you fly—the less air in the sky."

The point should be quite clear. Above 10,000 feet, think oxygen. If you do not have oxygen, stay at the lower altitudes. (See Figures 2-7, 2-8, 2-9, and 2-10.) For you turbo jockeys, note that

Figure 2-6.
This table demonstrates the relationship of the alveolar, or lung oxygen, to the blood oxygen saturation. Note that once we achieve an altitude of greater than 10,000 feet, our blood oxygen saturation drops below 92%, which is where we run into trouble. This is exactly why oxygen is mandatory beyond 10,000 feet. Remember that our time of useful consciousness at 18,000 feet, assuming we are a nonsmoker, is only about 30 minutes.

Altitude	ALVEOLAR OXYGEN Partial Pressure	BLOOD OXYGEN Saturation
Sea Level	101 mm Hg.	97%
5,000 feet	82 mm Hg.	95%
10,000 feet	65 mm Hg.	92%
15,000 feet	60 mm Hg.	90%
20,000 feet	45 mm Hg.	80%
25,000 feet	35 mm Hg.	75%
30,000 feet	24 mm Hg.	47%
35,000 feet	14 mm Hg.	25%
40,000 feet	11 mm Hg.	15%

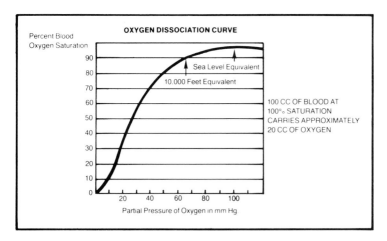

Figure 2-7.
A simple oxygen dissociation curve demonstrates that beyond 10,000 feet, oxygen blood saturation drops below 90%, which is the limit of tolerance in a healthy person for maximum performance.

ALTITUDE PRESSURE TABLE

ALTITUDE	PRESSURE	RATIO
Sea Level	760 mm Hg. – 14.7 psi	1 atmosphere
5,000 feet	633 mm Hg. – 12.2 psi	
10,000 feet	522 mm Hg. – 10.1 psi	
15,000 feet	429 mm Hg. – 8.3 psi	
18,000 feet	380 mm Hg. – 7.3 psi	½ atmosphere
20,000 feet	350 mm Hg. – 6.7 psi	
25,000 feet	282 mm Hg. – 5.5 psi	
27,000 feet	252 mm Hg. – 4.9 psi	⅓ atmosphere
30,000 feet	226 mm Hg. – 4.4 psi	
33,000 feet	196 mm Hg. – 3.8 psi	
35,000 feet	179 mm Hg. – 3.5 psi	¼ atmosphere
40,000 feet	141 mm Hg. – 2.7 psi	

Figure 2-8.
An altitude pressure table demonstrates the relationship of the altitude to the pressures in millimeters of mercury, which can be converted into psi to use in calculating cabin pressures. Notice that at 18,000 feet, one-half atmosphere, or 7.3 psi, is present in an ambient cabin without pressurization.

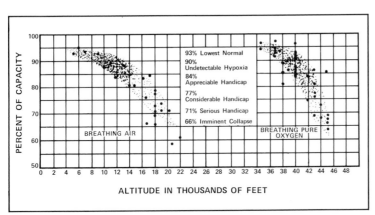

Figure 2-9.
Oxygen saturation (percent of capacity) of arterial blood and the range of performance at various altitudes in subjects breathing air and in subjects breathing oxygen. Note that performance diminishes markedly after 10,000 feet when breathing cabin air. On the other hand, 100% oxygen allows excellent function well above 30,000 feet. The message is clear. Use oxygen beyond 10,000 feet.

49

pushing above 40,000 feet without a pressurized airplane is a physical impossibility. Even on 100% oxygen, you will not receive an adequate supply to prevent hypoxia. A good suggestion for folks using supplemental oxygen is to go through the Air Force flight chamber briefing described earlier.

There are varying requirements for the nonsmoker and smoker. At 10,000 feet the nonsmoker, during the day, is a happy, contented, safe pilot. When the same nonsmoker ascends from 10,000 to 18,000 feet, he should initiate the use of oxygen (earlier at night). The smoker will, of course, require oxygen much earlier than the nonsmoker since he is already at a physiological 8,000 feet when he takes off at sea level. The real danger in the range from 10,000 to 18,000 feet is that the smoker will not notice hypoxia creeping

Figure 2-10.
Pulmonary gases at equivalent altitudes when breathing air or pure oxygen. Notice that the pressure of oxygen in the tracheal-inspired air provides for an adequate alveolar oxygen pressure of 10,000 feet on ambient, or cabin air, but to 40,000 feet while breathing pure oxygen. The advantage of having oxygen on board should be most clear.

EQUIVALENT ALTITUDES		BREATHING	TRACHEAL INSPIRED PO_2 mm Hg.	ALVEOLAR		R*
Feet	mm Hg.			PO_2 mm Hg.	PCO_2 mm Hg.	
Sea Level	760	air	149	103	40	.85
34,000	188	oxygen	141	101	40	
5,000	632	air	123	80	38	.87
36,500	167	oxygen	120	82	38	
10,000	523	air	100	61	36	0.90
39,500	145	oxygen	98	62	36	
15,000	429	air	80	46	33	0.95
42,000	128	oxygen	81	48	33	
18,000	380	air	70	38	31	0.98
44,000	117	oxygen	70	39	31	
20,000	350	air	64	34	30	1.00
45,000	111	oxygen	64	34	30	
22,000	321	air	57	30	28	1.05
46,000	106	oxygen	59	30	29	

* R = Respiratory Exchange Ratio (VCO_2/VO_2).

up on him; so his performance, both physically and mentally, will be degraded.

The oxygen dissociation curves for human blood are affected by the acidity (pH) of the blood. It tends to be a shift toward the right (that's bad) when the patient is acidic, or the pH in the blood has lowered. Such conditions can occur in diabetics, in people with gastrointestinal problems, and in people with chronic respiratory diseases. The point is that any oxygen dissociation curve is based on a healthy, normal individual. Better to err on the side of having a little more oxygen on board than not enough. Better to concern yourself with the state of health of your passengers and check with an AME before you take anybody with any sort of medical problem into an oxygen-requiring environment.

In the era of turbocharged small airplanes that are capable of ascending to positive control space altitudes, pilots must be cautious of their limitations to tolerate ambient oxygen conditions. The TUC (time of useful consciousness) following removal of oxygen at 24,000 feet is roughly two minutes. Simply put, if we do not rapidly find a source of oxygen either in an emergency supply or by descending, we have limited time before we are incapacitated. (See Figures 2-11 and 2-12.)

That the oxygen gradient from the blood to the lungs should become positive at higher altitudes suggests that at some point the body tissues, and in particular the brain, will not receive enough oxygen and, therefore, fail to function properly. This, in fact, happens. At 18,000 feet, the time of useful consciousness in the average pilot is 30 minutes, but decreases to 10 minutes at 22,000 feet and to four minutes at Flight Level 250. At 30,000 feet, you have only one minute of useful consciousness and at 40,000 feet, nine seconds, or roughly the time for the blood to circulate around the body once. If the altitude is achieved rapidly,

STAGES OF HYPOXIA

| STAGE | ALTITUDE IN FEET | | ARTERIAL OXYGEN SATURATION % |
	Breathing Air	Breathing 100% Oxygen	
Indifferent	0 to 10,000	34,000 to 39,000	95 to 90
Compensatory	10,000 to 15,000	39,000 to 42,500	90 to 80
Disturbance	15,000 to 20,000	42,500 to 44,800	80 to 70
Critical	20,000 to 23,000	44,800 to 45,500	70 to 60

Figure 2-11

lists the stages of hypoxia: indifferent, compensatory, disturbance, and critical. Notice as you look at the column of "altitude in feet" that our hypoxia resistance is much greater breathing 100% oxygen. Notice, however, that beyond 40,000 feet something more than 100% oxygen is needed. This something more is pressure breathing. Unless we have special equipment, such as in experimental or military aircraft, we have no business at these altitudes. Looking at the breathing-air column, we can appreciate that beyond 15,000 feet, even in general aviation craft, we must employ oxygen to avoid hypoxia. As a matter of fact, we really should use oxygen at any altitude over 10,000 feet and even earlier at night. As you might expect, the arterial oxygen saturation, which is the real bottom line in hypoxia, diminishes markedly above 10,000 feet when we are breathing air or above 39,000 feet when we are breathing 100% oxygen. When we are working with less than 90% arterial oxygen saturation, we are potentially in trouble.

such as in a decompression when a bomb goes off inside a 707, the time of useful consciousness is roughly halved. The time of useful consciousness in smokers is roughly half that of nonsmokers. It makes you think about how fast you would have to reach for that dangling oxygen mask if you suddenly decompressed a passenger plane at Flight Level 380. It does indeed provide incentive to move a mite rapidly.

Hypemic Hypoxia is more common than you think. The hypemic portion refers to diminished useful hemoglobin, which is responsible for binding the oxygen in the red blood cells. The most obvious cause of diminished hemoglobin is anemia, either secondary to bleeding or low iron, or inability to absorb the nutrients responsible for manufacturing hemoglobin.[1] In a healthy patient population, the most predisposing factor for loss of blood would probably be donating blood. This is why the military services will not allow their pilots to fly for 72 hours after making a blood donation. Technicalities notwithstanding, the most common cause of hypemic hypoxia in our

---

[1] A genetic trait called sickle cell anemia, more often present in people of Mediterranean or African black descent, can manifest itself as hypemic hypoxia; sicklemia can be detected by blood testing.

private pilot population is decreased hemoglobin due to carbon monoxide binding. I don't mean to imply that all New York City residents will be more susceptible to hypoxia than those living in the hills of Maine (although this may be true). I do mean to imply that if you are a smoker, there is a good chance that 10% of your hemoglobin will be bound up with carbon monoxide. Since carbon monoxide has a greater affinity for hemoglobin than does oxygen, the hemoglobin thus becomes unavailable for oxygen. (See Figure 2-13.) To show you how dramatically smoking (your smoking friends can do it to you) can lead to hypoxia, witness the fact that three cigarettes or one cigar can reduce enough circulating hemoglobin to place you physiologically at an altitude

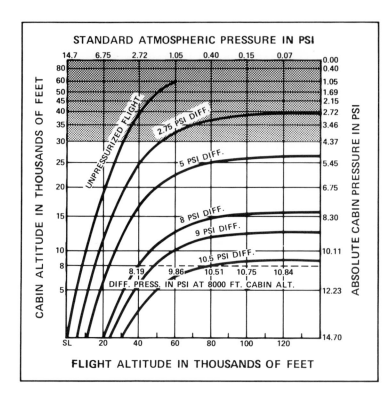

Figure 2-12 demonstrates cabin pressure schedules and physiological thresholds at various flight altitudes. Since most of us are dealing with unpressurized or low PSI differentials, we must shift our eyes to the left. It is important for us to realize that the time at which we can maintain high altitudes is a function of our cabin altitude. We must always anticipate loss of pressure, read our cabin pressure as part of our periodic checklist, and be prepared to descend immediately and/or don oxygen masks.

of 8,000 feet while you are on the ground. Thus, when you, the smoker, finally reach 10,000 feet, you are already behind the power curve. The only cure for carbon monoxide binding is a long period of time with no smoking. Since you can't accomplish this in 24 hours prior to flight, perhaps now is the time for you to throw your cigarettes away.

Stagnant Hypoxia, the third type of hypoxia, is due to diminished blood flow to the brain. The word *stagnant* implies stagnation of blood below the level of the heart. Such stagnation takes place when you are pulling G forces (e.g., 60-degree-bank turns), when you have your legs crossed, or when you are pressure breathing, as in many of the newer turbocharged small aircraft. Stagnant

Figure 2-13.
Symptoms that develop at various concentrations of carbon monoxide in the blood. These symptoms should be learned and watched for while flying aircraft. Carbon monoxide can readily enter the cockpit from a nose-heater in a twin-engine craft or from a leak in the manifold, where heat emanates in a single-engine craft.

SYMPTOMS THAT DEVELOP AT VARIOUS CONCENTRATIONS OF CARBON MONOXIDE IN THE BLOOD

CARBON MONOXIDE, PERCENT IN BLOOD	SYMPTOMS
0 to 10	None.
10 to 20	Tightness across forehead, possibly slight headache, dilatation of cutaneous blood vessels.
20 to 30	Headache, throbbing in temples.
30 to 40	Severe headache, weakness, dizziness, dimness of vision, nausea and vomiting, and collapse.
40 to 50	Same as previous, with increased pulse rate and respiration, and more possibility of collapse.
50 to 60	Syncope, increased respiration and pulse, coma with intermittent convulsions, Cheyne-Stokes type of respiration.
60 to 70	Coma with intermittent convulsions, depressed heart action—possibly death.
70 to 80	Weak pulse and slowed respiration, respiratory failure and death.

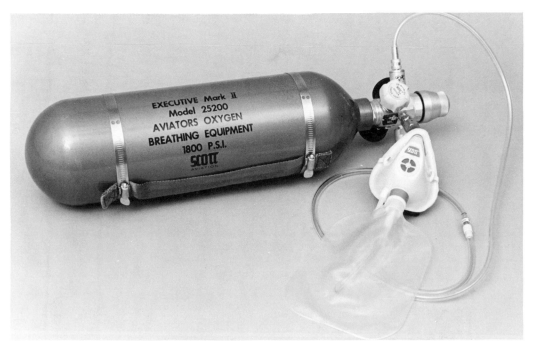

Figure 2-14
is a picture of a typical portable
oxygen system available for general
aviation aircraft. Any pilot employ-
ing oxygen should first attend an
FAA-sponsored flight chamber ride
in order to orient himself on hypoxia, hyperventilation, and proper
oxygen usage.
(Courtesy Scott Aviation)

hypoxia is less likely to affect private pilots who
are healthy. Should you be flying on a waiver for
poor circulation and/or a condition that allows
blood pooling, you are probably aware that you
will be more susceptible to stagnant hypoxia.

Histotoxic Hypoxia is the fourth type of hypoxia. As the name implies, tissues *(histo)* become
toxic from some outside drug (e.g., cyanide),
which blocks the tissue uptake of oxygen even
though it might be present in the blood in
normal quantities. A most common blocker is
alcohol. We will discuss alcohol a great deal
because of its common occurrence in pilots who
suffer fatal accidents. Perhaps less well understood is that a small amount of alcohol, while
having no significant hypoxic effects at sea level,
is markedly potentiated at altitude. The two
drinks with which you safely drove home after
your office party last Friday night can be fatal at

OXYGEN DURATION IN HOURS AND MINUTES

Control Setting At Altitude	NO. OF MASKS IN USE			
	1	2	3	4
8-12	6:10	2:50	1:56	1:30
12-16	4:56	2:28	1:35	1:08
16-20	3:53	1:50	1:16	0:54
20-25	3:06	1:30	0:58	0:42
25-30	2:30	1:12	0:48	0:36

Durations are approximate and are based on full cylinder starting pressure of 1800 PSIG with portable at altitude indicated. Durations will be less if portable is used at ground level.

Figure 2-15.
It is important that you understand the duration of your oxygen supply under a variety of circumstances. This is a typical oxygen-duration table for portable general aviation equipment.
(Courtesy Puritan Bennett Aero Systems Company)

8,000 feet. Remember, the tissue toxic effect of alcohol exceeds the time over which it is metabolized and excreted. The rule of "eight hours from bottle to throttle" may work in the day and at low altitudes. You can be pushing your luck at night and at higher altitudes if you don't allow an even longer period of time. The current military policy, therefore, is to allow 24 hours of drying out.

Hypoxia Treatment

The best treatment for hypoxia is, of course, prevention. Learn to recognize symptoms early; maintain, preflight, and use your O_2 equipment properly. Avoid hypoxic hypoxia by not flying when you are ill (e.g., pneumonia), and don't fly above 10,000 feet without using supplemental oxygen (see Figures 2-14, 2-15 and 2-16). Avoid hypemic hypoxia by not flying after donating blood or after an injury with a significant blood loss; use oxygen earlier in the game if you're foolish enough to continue smoking. Avoid histotoxic hypoxia by not flying for at least 24 hours after you have been drinking; and don't fly while

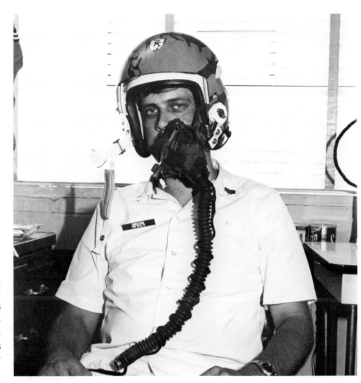

Figure 2-16
shows a form-fitting oxygen
mask with a close-fitting head
set and protective helmet as
employed by the military. Because most civilian oxygen
masks do not fit as well as this
example, a high oxygen flow
should be maintained.

on medication without the approval of an AME.
Prevention notwithstanding, the treatment is
clear: should hypoxia appear, descend and add
oxygen! If you don't have oxygen aboard, descend! Descend as rapidly as is safely possible!
Oh, for a set of speed brakes on a 172!

PRICE Check

Those of you fortunate enough to go through
an FAA flight chamber will be exposed to a
PRICE check. PRICE is the acronym used for
checking oxygen equipment. PRICE is to oxygen
as GUMP (Gas, Undercarriage, Mixture, Prop) is
to landing. PRICE is an acronym for Pressure,
Regulator, Indicator, Connections, Emergency: 1.
Pressure tells you to make sure you have oxygen

on board by checking the pressure gauge on the tank; make certain you have enough for the flight time projected. 2. *Regulator* means to check the unit for over-all conditions; make sure that the settings are proper and that your diaphragm (if you have one) is working properly. 3. *Indicator*, of course, should be on, and should demonstrate that there is a good flow and that an adequate seal can be made around your oxygen mask. If you do have a breathing indicator, it is also a good measure of rate of breathing to tip you off to hyperventilation. 4. *Connections* should be checked to make sure that they are intact, not leaking, and are clean. 5. The *Emergency* supply of oxygen should be that small amount tucked aside for your use in case disaster strikes.

Oxygen equipment is not different from any other equipment on the airplane; oxygen systems require conscientious preflight. When flying in a rarefied atmosphere, a **PRICE** check can be a lifesaver.

Hyperventilation

Hyperventilation can be confused with hypoxia and is, therefore, important to understand. Hyperventilation is derived from *hyper,* meaning too much or too great, and *ventilation,* meaning breathing. Hyperventilation is, therefore, too great a rate or depth of breathing. This blows off carbon dioxide from the lungs.

The resulting symptoms of hyperventilation are very similar to those of hypoxia. The pilot is frequently dizzy, faint, may be tingling, numb, or cool, and sometimes experiences hot and cold flashes. The key symptom of hyperventilation that distinguishes the symptom complex from hypoxia is *muscle spasm.* The hypoxic person is relaxed and his muscles flabby; the pilot with severe hyperventilation is tense and his muscles are in spasm.

The cause of hyperventilation is usually anxiety, even when the pilot may not be aware that he is anxious. Flying IFR around a thunderstorm can be anxiety-producing, but so can your first solo flight. Sometimes anxiety overcomes even the most experienced pilots and under not very trying circumstances.

The treatment is simple. Relax! Slow down the rate and depth of your breathing. Since it may be difficult to distinguish hypoxia from hyperventilation, switch to 100% oxygen if you have oxygen equipment on board.

To prevent hyperventilation, recognize an increased rate of breathing. If you find yourself pumping your lungs away and breathing rapidly, hold your breath, slow down the rate of your breathing, and relax.

Hyperventilation can be remembered with the acronym FAST. FAST stands for Fear, Anxiety, Stress, and Tension, which are the primary causes of hyperventilation. Although we may be unaware of the causes, the rapid breathing of hyperventilation blows off carbon dioxide, and leads to lightheadedness and giddiness, which we may misinterpret as hypoxia. Hyperventilation can be controlled with slow, even breathing and if necessary, by breathing into a bag to increase the carbon dioxide level in our blood.

Ozone Sickness

Ozone sickness was not well recognized until the mid to late 1970s. Standards to control ozone levels in high-flying airplanes were implemented in 1981.

Ozone is a toxic variant of the normal oxygen molecule. Oxygen consists of two oxygen atoms hooked together to form the oxygen molecule. It is this normal O_2 that comprises approximately 20 percent of the atmosphere we breathe. It is the absence of this O_2 in our tissues that accounts for hypoxia. When a single oxygen atom is hooked to the normal O_2 molecule, creating a three-atom oxygen molecule (O_3), the molecule is called ozone. Ozone is very unstable and tends to break down into normal, breathable oxygen and free oxygen atoms. Ozone exists in relatively high levels at altitudes above 35,000 feet. Since most airplanes did not fly at these altitudes until the introduction of high-altitude jets, the effects of ozone have been slow to be recognized. Because jet streams and aircraft efficiency are increased at high levels, much of our intercontinental and transcontinental airline travel now takes place at altitudes of relatively high ozone concentration. The ozone layer tends to be in a higher concentration during January through May. The total concentration is highly variable and is markedly elevated in some years, for as-yet poorly understood reasons. Ozone is more common in northern latitudes.

Symptoms of ozone sickness generate multiple complaints including chest pains, a deep hacking cough, eye irritation similar to that caused by smog, bloody and running noses, and difficulty with breathing. Symptoms were first described by flight attendants in 1977. Because of multiple complaints from flight attendants and pilots, the FAA initiated a series of studies at its Civil Aeromedical Institute in Oklahoma City. During these initial studies, they exposed 83 people in an altitude chamber to a variety of ozone levels. Physicians could demonstrate restriction of airflow into the lungs, usually starting at levels of 0.2 to 0.3 parts ozone per million. Subsequent measurements by the National Aeronautic and Space Administration on high-level flights on

several different airlines found levels of one part
ozone per million, or more than five times the
level that the FAA had demonstrated would cause
symptoms.

The FAA therefore instituted a regulation, the
compliance deadline for which was February 20,
1981. The regulation requires an average ozone
level not to exceed 0.1 ozone parts per million for
long-range flights, with all peaks required to be
less than 0.25 parts ozone per million. This 10-
fold reduction in ozone from the ambient environment to the plane's interior environment can
be accomplished by a variety of methods. Char-
coal filters have been found effective. The char-
coal filters adequate to reduce ozone levels in, say,
a 747 weigh approximately 600 pounds. Because
of the high weight load, the carrying capacity of
the airplane must be reduced. Therefore, airlines
are currently switching to catalytic converters,
which are currently being supplied by Lockheed
in its L-1011 jets and by Boeing in its current 747
and 747SP jets. Estimates by the FAA suggest that
filters in some 500 United States jets will cost
somewhere between seven and 12 million dollars,
so a great deal of funding is needed to control
ozone levels. Such control will, we hope, reduce
the apparently transient problem of potentially
severe symptoms of ozone sickness.

Trapped Gas and Pressure Change

As we can well imagine, any gas that is trapped
in any space in your body will tend to increase in
volume as the pressure around it decreases. It's
the old balloon trick except it's inside you. A gas
volume of one will increase two-fold at 16,000
feet, five-fold at 34,000 feet, and seven-fold at

Figure 2-17 demonstrates the theoretical expansion of internal body gases upon equalization with a variety of cabin differential pressures from one through eight psi. The important fact to be culled from this graph is that our internal body cavity gases will expand as we ascend in altitude, almost regardless of the pressure differential we maintain in our cabin. In view of those of us operating non-pressurized and pressurized general aviation craft in higher altitudes, it is important for us to remember the old adage, poop and burp. We must encourage our passengers to do the same to maintain comfort.

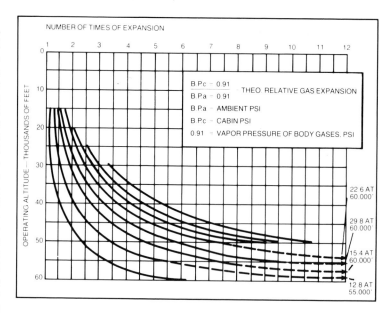

39,000 feet. If you don't release the gas, you become the balloon (see Figure 2-17).

The Bowels

When the stomach and intestines are involved, release is usually easy. As you ascend through the atmosphere and the pressure around you decreases, the gas that has expanded inside your body is released. If your bowels are a problem, avoid fast eating and gas-producing foods such as soda pop, cabbage, beans, and spicy foods. To relieve the pressure is a necessity. Avoid chewing gum while ascending, since air swallowing may occur. In the case of air-containing cavities such as the middle ear, sinus, and pockets in your teeth, release may not be simple.

The Sinus and Ear

An increase in altitude is associated with escape of air from the sinus and/or middle ear space (see

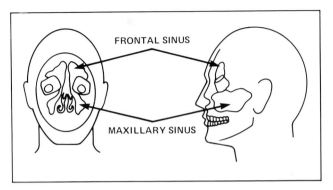

FRONTAL SINUS

MAXILLARY SINUS

Figure 2-18
demonstrates the paranasal sinuses. The sinuses serve to keep the skull strong and light. These air-filled cavities within the bones of the face are subject to blockage from colds. The two major sinuses above and below the eyes, respectively, are the frontal and maxillary sinuses. It is these sinuses that can become blocked on descent and lead to severe, incapacitating pain.

Figure 2-18). In the case of the sinus, air is expelled into the nose involuntarily. In the case of the ear, air is expelled into the back of the nose by way of the eustachian tube—sometimes you can hear an audible click or feel the pressure released as this air escape takes place. On descent, the air pressure around you increases, and it is necessary to replace the air in your sinus or ear. Should the

Figure 2-19
illustrates the mechanism of fluid and pain formation in the sinus during flight. If we follow the sinus (be it maxillary or frontal—see Figure 2-18) from left to right, we can note the pressure changes. The sinus at sea level may have a small residual fluid level in it. Our total sinuses produce 1.5 pints of fluid a day, which we swallow and is no cause for concern. As we ascend, the positive pressure in the sinus relative to the lesser pressure in the air around us, pushes air out of the sinus. We may even hear this as an audible click. However, as we descend, air must return into the sinus to equilibrate the pressure. If the sinus entrance into the nose is blocked by a cold, allergy or tumor, air cannot re-enter the sinus, and a negative pressure develops. To fill this negative pressure, fluid accumulates in the sinus and/or we suddenly bleed into the sinus. This leads to acute, incapacitating pain. If a sinus block occurs, do not continue your descent. Re-ascend and spray your nose with a decongestant medication, which you should always carry in your flight kit. After allowing enough time for the medication to take effect (say three to four minutes), try a gentle descent again. If a sinus block and/or pain develop, you should surely see your physician after you land.

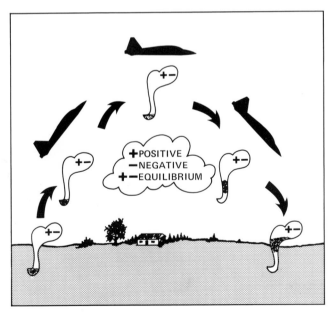

+ POSITIVE
− NEGATIVE
+ − EQUILIBRIUM

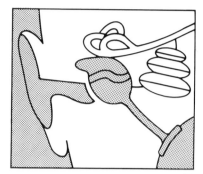

Increased barometric pressure
on an unventilated middle ear
(during descent).

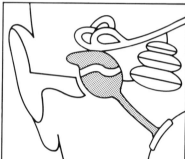

Decreased barometric pressure
on an unventilated middle ear
(during ascent).

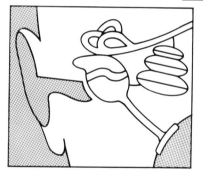

Sea Level—middle ear pressure
equal to that of the atmosphere.

Figure 2-20

demonstrates the pressure relations between the middle ear and the
flying environment. At sea level, the ear is in equilibrium with the
surrounding environment. During ascent, we enter a rarefied atmosphere, and pressure builds within the middle ear. Air bubbles from
the middle ear through the eustachian tube into the back of the nose.
We sometimes hear this as a click. During descent, however, pressure
builds in the environment, and we must move air into our middle ear
to equalize the pressure. If the eustachian tube is blocked by a cold or
other disease, this may not be achieved. Negative pressure can result
in pain, eardrum or tympanic membrane rupture, and/or in vertigo.

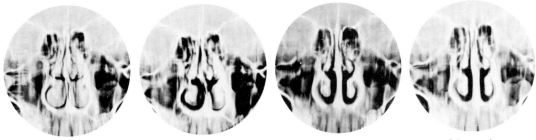

| Pretreatment | 5 minutes later | 4 hours later | 12 hours later |

passage to your sinus or ear block up, as with a cold or too rapid a descent, inflammation and subsequent bleeding into the sinus or ear may take place. In the case of the sinus, the pain may become so incapacitating and the headache so severe that the pilot is unable to control his aircraft (see Figures 2-19 and 2-20). In the case of the middle ear, the pain may be compounded by hearing loss and instant vertigo, which is equally incapacitating. The solution is obvious. First, don't fly with a head cold or with any form of nasal obstruction. Second, chew gum while descending, hold your nose and swallow to clear your ears and sinuses, and avoid rapid descent.

Should an ear or sinus block occur, reascend. Then spray your nose with a local decongestant such as Afrin (see Figure 2-21). A local decongestant should be carried in your flight bag. Allow three or four minutes for the medication to take effect and try descending again. Take it slowly, with a lot of swallowing.

Should you be continually unsuccessful in clearing your ears or sinuses, see your AME or ear, nose, and throat physician immediately. It is possible that medication prescribed by the physician may resolve your problem. It may be necessary to equalize the pressure in your middle ear with a myringotomy, or hole in the eardrum, to avoid a permanent hearing problem and/or infection. It may be necessary to drain any blood or

Figure 2-21
demonstrates the effect of a long-acting nasal decongestant spray such as Afrin. The xeroradiographs demonstrate the effect of the nasal spray on the mucous membranes within the nasal cavity. The view is taken from front to back and shows the large curlicue tissue structure (turbinates), which, when swollen, obstruct the sinuses. These swollen turbinates account for not only a feeling of nasal obstruction but also for the inability of the sinus to equilibrate as the ambient pressure changes. Within minutes after being sprayed, the mucous membranes of the turbinates shrink, allowing for both better breathing and adequate aeration of the sinuses. Whenever a sinus block occurs during flying, the nose should be sprayed with a decongestant while the pilot is reascending. One should not continue a descent when a sinus or ear block occurs.

Figure 2-22
represents the normal tympanic membrane or eardrum through which the ossicles (ear bones) can be seen. The ossicles occupy the middle ear space, transmitting the sound from the eardrum to the neural structures of the inner ear. When these ossicles are dampened by fluid, they cannot conduct vibration properly, and hearing loss results.

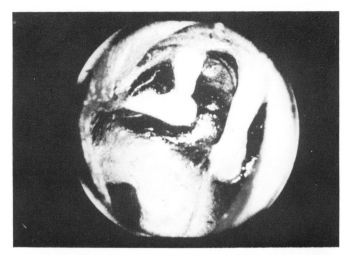

Figure 2-23
shows a serous effusion behind the eardrum which has resulted from inadequate eustachian tube function or a failure by the pilot to clear his ears. Upon descent, swallow to open the tube and equalize the pressure in the middle ear. If negative pressure persists within the middle ear, fluid accumulates to equalize the pressure.

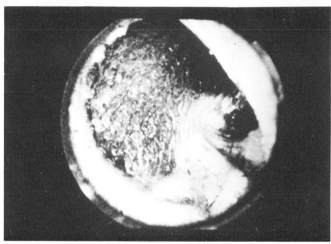

Figure 2-24
shows a perforation or hole within the eardrum caused by the pilot's failure to equalize the pressure within his middle ear. In this case, when pain arose on descent, the pilot did not stop the descent and/or equalize the pressure within his middle ear space. The negative pressure became great enough to rupture the eardrum.

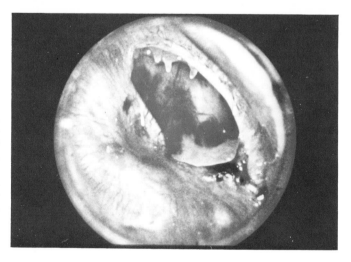

fluid that is sucked into your sinus before a further problem occurs. (See Figures 2-22, 2-23, 2-24, and 2-25.) One way or the other, you should not attempt to treat the delicate structures of your ear or sinus by yourself. This is a clear-cut case of your need for a doctor.

Decompression Sickness

Decompression sickness is caused by gases evolving within the body due to reduced pressure of the atmosphere. Decompression sickness need not necessarily occur at a very high altitude. Decompression sickness has been reported as low as 5,000 feet, by pilots who have recently been scuba diving. Let's look at the underlying reasons for decompression sickness, some of the symptoms, how to prevent it, and how to treat it.

As we know, the air around us exerts a pressure of 760 millimeters of mercury. Eighty percent of this air is made up of nitrogen. When you place pressure on air overlying fluid, air or gas is forced into the fluid. A carbonated beverage is made using this principle. But that same bottle of soda, when the cap is released, releases gas. If your body tissues are the can of soda, and you suddenly decrease the pressure around you, gas in your body can similarly bubble out. Since the gas around us is 80 percent nitrogen, and since most of the oxygen is bound to hemoglobin, it is the nitrogen that bubbles out.

Symptoms

The nitrogen can bubble into the joints, creating extreme pain and doubling the pilot over. This is called the "bends" because the body goes into a bent position due to the pain. The nitrogen can bubble out under the skin, producing an itch,

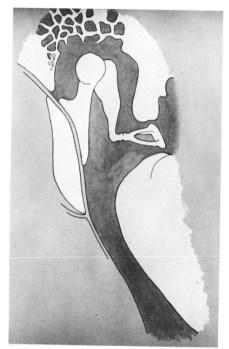

A

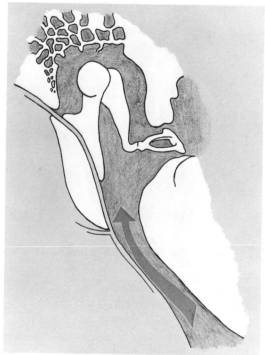

B

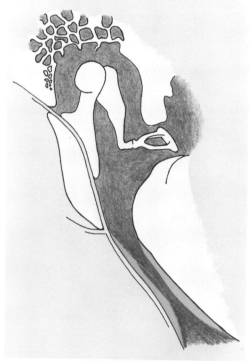

C

Figure 2-25

shows a cross section of the middle ear space. On the left (A) is the eardrum connected to the first ear-bone (malleus) and thence through the second and third ear-bones, the incus and the stapes, or stirrup, to the inner ear on the right. The middle ear space pressure is equalized by the eustachian tube, which extends from the middle ear space down more vertically into the nose. As can be seen by the arrow in B, air must enter the eustachian tube to equalize the negative pressure on descent. In C, if the eustachian tube is blocked (by disease, a cold, or failure to swallow), negative pressure will develop. When this happens, as seen in D, fluid accumulates

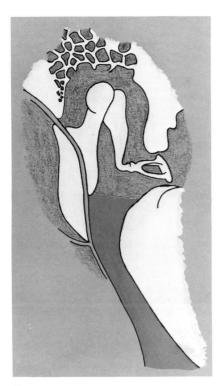

D

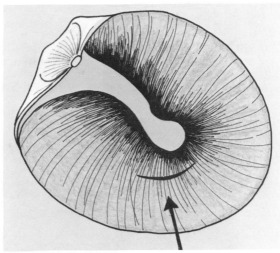

E

in the middle ear. Should this fluid not be cleared by decongestant sprays, it may be necessary to perform a myringotomy or paracentesis (E). Following this paracentesis, a small needle suction, as seen in F, is employed for clearing the fluid out of the middle ear space. The tiny hole in the eardrum then heals itself. The pilot will have no subsequent hearing loss.
(Courtesy Richards Manufacturing Company, Inc.)

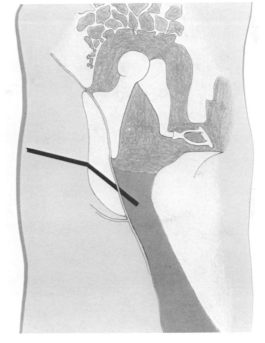

F

a tingling sensation, little electric-like pulses, or even a rash. The nitrogen can bubble out into the lungs, causing a choking sensation, difficulty in breathing, and a dry, hacking cough. It is possible for so much air to be introduced into the circulatory system that a bolus, or collection of bubbles, is sent up to the brain, where a stroke-like pattern occurs, sometimes leaving the pilot unconscious. Finally, the nitrogen can bubble out into the central nervous system itself, producing loss of vision, motor weakness, weird sensations, or loss of mental capacity and even unconsciousness.

So, decompression sickness is symptomatically a spectrum ranging from an itch on the skin to mild or severe joint pains, to a choking or inability to gain your breath, all the way to a complete central nervous system collapse. It is a symptom complex, therefore, not to be disregarded.

Cause

Decompression sickness, following a sudden loss of pressure around us, can occur in a pressurized aircraft where a leak suddenly develops. But the average private pilot is most likely to have decompression sickness as a result of a gradual ascent into a rarefied environment. If he has been scuba diving, he is much more prone to decompression sickness. Each 33 feet of water is equal to one atmosphere (760 millimeters mercury) pressure. So, if he has been down 50 or 60 feet, or two atmospheres, the pilot has already had nitrogen pushed into body tissues. This nitrogen is just waiting to bubble out when he ascends even into a relatively low altitude. A word to the wise—wait 24 hours after scuba diving before flying, or fly *very* low!

TREATMENT

Given symptoms of decompression sickness, what can you do?

DESCEND. Get your butt down and now. If you have 100 percent oxygen, use it. Even if your symptoms disappear after descending, see a doctor. The decompression sickness can be just starting, can be relieved for a while, and can recur while on the ground, with fatal results. What you are going to need is a compression chamber.

Once you have landed and have seen your AME, he will send you to the nearest military or civilian pressure chamber, where you will be placed in a 100% oxygen environment and taken down (pressurized) to a below-sea-level altitude (see Figure 2-26). Eventually, step-by-step, you will be brought back up to sea level when your physicians are certain all nitrogen has been washed from your body tissues. This sounds like a lot to go through for a symptom complex that might not be severe. True—but it can also save your life.

TEMPERATURE and SURVIVAL

Temperature is a very important consideration for pilots in terms of their flying environment and their potential survival environment. Consider that the earth's surface temperature ranges from –90° F to +140° F, changing with time and place in a horizontal mode. Over a vertical displacement from the earth's crust, we have learned that the adiabatic lapse rate approaches approximately 3° F per 1,000 feet, degrees which we subtract as we ascend. So, if the temperature

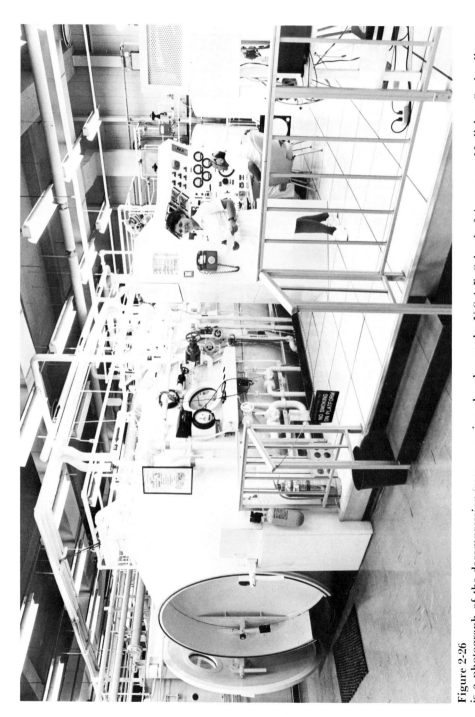

Figure 2-26
is a photograph of the decompression/recompression chamber at the U.S.A.F. School of Aerospace Medicine. Scuba divers and/or other pilots subjected to rapid decompression, who subsequently develop the bends or evidence of neurological sequelae, are immediately transported to a similar recompression chamber. Pressure is again built up. Patients are placed on 100% oxygen, and (following denitrogenation) altitude is decreased slowly to sea level, allowing the patient to recover. (Courtesy Col. Jefferson C. Davis)

outside is 60° F on takeoff, after climbing 6,000 feet, we expect the temperature to be approximately 40° F. The temperature throughout the troposphere, the lower level of the atmosphere in which we fly, is highly variable. Regardless of how we look at it, as we ascend, the temperature usually decreases. Maintaining our aircraft cabins within limits of a comfortable temperature is important. When we are either too cold or too hot, our performance decreases just like an airplane's—we perform best in low humidity and moderate temperatures. The thermal requirements for human tolerance are laid out in Figure 2-27. Note that the comfort zone is a relatively small area of 65°-95° F.

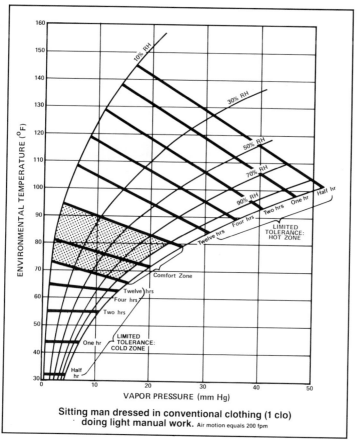

Sitting man dressed in conventional clothing (1 clo) doing light manual work. Air motion equals 200 fpm

Figure 2-27.
Thermal requirements for our aircraft cockpits have been well delineated by extensive experimentation. The comfort zone is fairly clearly defined between 65° and 95°F as a function of time and circulation. The message in this graph is that maximum pilot performance, both physically and mentally, is a function of proper temperature and humidity. Keep in mind that we can push ourselves just so far. We are much better off maintaining a maximum comfort zone, which will better our performance in the cockpit.

Heat can be lost in one of four ways: conduction, convection, radiation, and evaporation. The important thing for pilots to remember is that there is little they can do to control those four processes except to wear comfortable clothing and use the airplane heaters and/or vent system as best they can to maintain a comfort level. You can get some idea of the limits of tolerance as related to performance by looking at Figure 2-28. It is important that a pilot not push himself to the limits of tolerance, but be aware of the effects of temperature and its degradation on both mental and physical performance. Above and beyond its recognition, the best way to handle temperature extremes is to be in good physical condition.

Figure 2-28 demonstrates that the limits of body performance in extreme temperature are not confined to degradation in cold temperature. Excessive heat makes it difficult for us to function as well. Note that as we move beyond one hour in extreme temperatures, very few of us can perform useful tasks. The message here is to keep our cockpits as cool as possible. Make sure we have maximum air circulating through the cockpit. Take time to cool off if it is impossible to cool the cockpit down adequately.

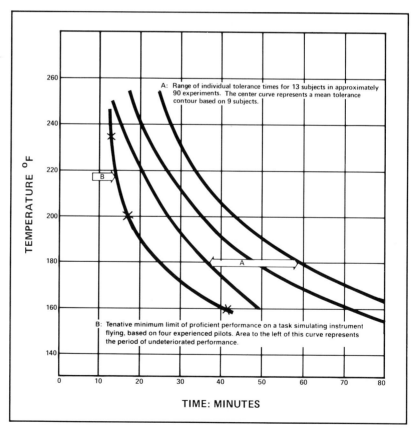

Of primary concern to every aviation pilot is the effect temperature will have on him should he not land on an airfield. I once had an instructor in Southern California who would not fly with me unless I brought along a jacket and gloves in case we ever decided to land in the mountains. Not a bad idea! Some of the fatalities in general aviation accidents are caused not by the crash itself but by the inability of the occupants to survive their environment after they arrive (usually unwillingly). Refer to Figures 2-29 and 2-30

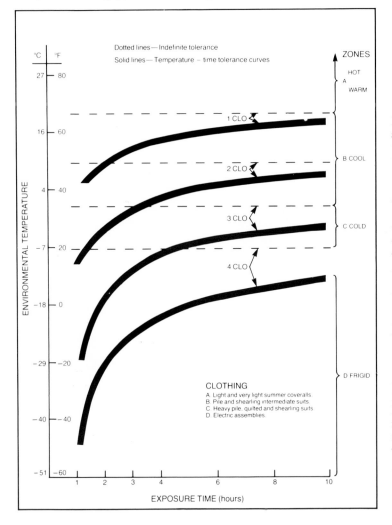

Figure 2-29 shows a series of cold tolerance curves under a variety of clothing (CLO) situations. The product to be extrapolated from this chart is that our exposure time in hours is markedly diminished at both cold *and* hot temperatures if our clothing is not appropriate. The most important conclusion to be drawn from these data is that clothing in your airplane should be appropriate for the weather conditions over which you are flying. Many general aviation craft accidents result in fatalities which would not have occurred if the victims had been able to walk away from the accident scene. An intelligent start to assure your survival is to have the proper clothing on board for survival in the worst possible climate to which you may be exposed.

Figure 2-30 demonstrates the wind-chill factors. The calorie demand or the amount of heat our bodies must generate increases dramatically as the velocity or miles per hour of the wind increases from zero to three or four. The excess calorie demand is more pronounced as the layers of clothing are decreased. The difference between having one layer of clothing and no layers of clothing, of course, is dramatic. You can appreciate that the more clothing you have in a windy situation, the better will be your protection against heat loss.

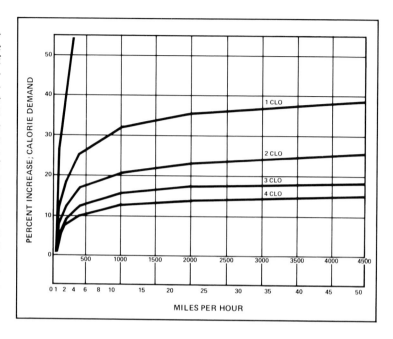

to appreciate how important extra clothing is for surviving in a cold environment. The case cannot be overstated for having appropriate survival gear on board for the area over which you are flying. No less is true of flying over cold water. See Figure 2-31 to appreciate that your survival in cold water is rapidly diminished as the temperature drops off. Experiments by the Germans in World War II showed that in ice water, the average man had only four or five minutes to get onto a secure platform or he would drown. This ought to give you an incentive to move right along should you go down in the North Atlantic Ocean, and you have something onto which you

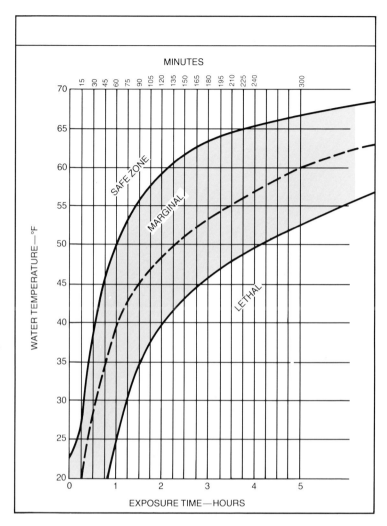

MINUTES

WATER TEMPERATURE—°F

SAFE ZONE

MARGINAL

LETHAL

EXPOSURE TIME—HOURS

Figure 2-31 demonstrates the short period of time during which we can tolerate cold water temperatures. Cold water acts as a heat draw on the body. If we were to land in the Atlantic Ocean during the winter, we would find the water temperatures slightly above freezing. If you look at the dot in the figure, you will see that after 30 minutes, the chances of surviving are slim. In fact, if we do not climb into a raft or some sort of floatable material in a matter of four to five minutes, the chances of our being able to do so are negligible.

can climb (a raft is preferable). Whether it is over desert, over snow, or over water, think survival and come prepared to encounter the thermal extremes of your environment.

CHAPTER 3

FORMS of DISORIENTATION

Spatial Disorientation

Spatial disorientation may be defined as lack of perception or appreciation of one's position in reference to the earth's surface. Spatial disorientation can be critical for pilots since disorientation can result in a fatal accident if immediate correction is not instituted by the pilot. Disorientation can occur in any pilot, regardless of his or her experience level. It is part of routine briefings in the Air Force for pilots who have many thousands of flying hours; it is part of refresher courses in flight chambers where a spatial disorientation trainer is frequently present. You should know not only that spatial disorientation can occur, but how to handle it.

THREE BASIC SENSES

There are three basic senses of equilibrium on which humans depend. 1. The *visual* (or ocular) sense is the primary mode of orientation during flying. 2. The *vestibular* (or inner ear) apparatus is invaluable on the earth's surface, but frequently fails as a primary means in the air; the semicircular canals and otolith organs make up the vestibular apparatus. 3. The *proprioceptive* (kinesthetic) or seat-of-the-pants sense may be valuable in performing certain acrobatic maneuvers, but is of little use to a disoriented pilot. Believe the first, or visual sense, by believing your aircraft instruments. Everything else lies. Let's take a look at the types of disorientation you can experience and the conditions under which disorientation most commonly occurs.

The vast majority of aircraft accidents are pilot induced. The single largest cause of fatal accidents is unusual attitudes and uncontrollable conditions as a direct result of disorientation in the pilot. It is, therefore, critical that we appreciate disorientation as soon as it occurs, and know how to handle it properly. Disorientation is most likely to be encountered on a dark night or in bad weather, or in borderline instrument flight conditions. When the real horizon is obscured, conditions for disorientation are ripe. Disorientation tends to be more common in less experienced pilots and in those whose instrument proficiency has slipped. Changing back and forth from the external environment to instrument flight has a tendency to produce disorientation. The resulting disorientation under the above circumstances can take many forms.

Vestibular Illusions

Forms of spatial disorientation are reported as: 1. leans; 2. somatogyral illusions; 3. oculogyral illusions; 4. Coriolis illusions; and 5. somatogravic illusions. These are all vestibular illusions.

1. The leans are classically exemplified in the pilot who is flying parallel to a slanted cloud bank but feels he is straight and level. The leans, therefore, result from an unperceived roll.

2. Somatogyral illusions are characterized by graveyard spirals. The sensation of direction that the pilot experiences is very different from the actual motion of the airplane.

3. The oculogyral illusion is characterized by return from the exterior environment to the instrument panel, at which point the panel appears to move, a clear-cut case of inner ear semicircular canal stimulation.

4. The Coriolis effect is an effect most readily perceived in the spatial disorientation trainer. When the pilot moves his head through a plane after the inner ear fluid is already rotating in a particular direction, marked disorientation occurs. You may have experienced this effect when turning to final and looking down to change a radio or view an instrument. The disorientation is marked and almost incapacitating.

5. The somatogravic illusion is caused by a perceived stimulation, as when power is applied and the airplane is rotated. The pilot feels as if he is climbing more than he is, lowers his nose, and ends up in full-power, shallow-angle collision beyond the end of the runway.

All of these forms of spatial disorientation are caused by an inner ear that is best suited to ground function. As you can see from Figure 5-9 on page 149, the three semicircular canals are designed to appreciate linear acceleration in the three different planes. This may be all right when your feet are on the ground; but when you are flying in an airplane, do not believe this sense. Believe your airplane's instrument gyro. The otolith organs on the other hand, as seen in Figure 5-8 on page 148, measure the pull of gravity. They do not do well when placed in a configuration different from standing upright with your feet on the ground. Do not believe them either. Believe your aircraft instrument gyro.

Visual Illusions

Visual illusions in the flying environment may be described as autokinesis and circular or linear-vection. *Autokinesis* is the illusion of a small light moving after you have stared at it in the dark for several seconds. At some point, you are not sure whether you are moving, the light is moving, or in which direction either is going. The solution is simple. Look at your gauges and buy what they tell you. *Circular-vection* is an illusion brought on by patterns coming into view from your eye's periphery. These create a false sense of rotation, in which case they are called circular-vection, or a false sense of linear movement, in which case the illusion is called linear-vection. Come back to the gauges and believe what they say. Remember that your visual sense is the sense most acutely affected by hypoxia. At night, even the young, healthy flier will have a 25 percent reduction in visual acuity at 8,000 feet and a 50 percent reduction in visual acuity at 12,000 feet. As seen in Figure 5-1 on page 125, one way to bring the rods, or the parts of the eye that are responsible for good night vision, into their best use is to scan. Flying at night is instrument flying at its best. Keep the head still and the eyes moving.

The perils of spatial disorientation cannot be appreciated more dramatically than by listening to a tape, from the FAA control tower archives, of the last moments of a military fighter pilot who, on a clear night, became disoriented while contacting center:

PILOT: Center, I have an instrument problem.
CENTER: State your problem.
PILOT: My instruments show a dive with my left wing down.
CENTER: Are you descending?
PILOT: Affirmative.
CENTER: Are you in a spin?
PILOT: I think so.
CENTER: Let your stick go, release back pressure, and apply opposite rudder.
PILOT: It's going the other way. It's going the other way.
CENTER: Release back pressure. Release your stick. I say, again, release your stick. Let the plane fly itself out.
PILOT: . . . .

That was the last transmission. The pilot was a 3,000-hour pilot with combat experience. The autopsy showed no physical incapacitations. We have all heard, and those of us in the crash investigation business have all seen, that no one is immune to spatial disorientation. Think of it, brief it to yourself, be prepared to counter it by believing your instruments and depending upon your flight training.

TREATMENT

The treatment for spatial disorientation is three-fold. The first is to recognize it. Do not panic, do not worry about it; admit disorientation and do something about it. The "do something about it" is looking at the gauges and believing in them. Remember that the white or light portion of the altitude gyro always belongs on top. Stupid, you say? I had a man flying my wing in formation who told me over the intercom that he was disoriented. When I looked over, he was flying perfect formation—inverted. He never knew it. The white belongs on top, I say again. Finally, instrument proficiency is a must. You cannot correct what you cannot do well. The man who thinks he is going to become instrument proficient as he plans an instrument flight is heading for spatial disorientation and a disaster. Think about it. Recognize disorientation; get on the gauges; stay instrument proficient.

Motion Sickness

Motion sickness has been experienced by most pilots during or after their training. The vast majority of Air Force student pilots have been motion sick at one point or another. A survey of over 300 experienced pilots showed that over 60 percent had been motion sick even after being certified. So, do not be ashamed if you are among the majority. Motion sickness is characterized by nausea, sweating, perhaps a headache, an uncomfortable feeling, and, occasionally, vomiting.

Vertigo

Vertigo is a term derived from the Latin *vertigo*, meaning "to turn." Vertigo is a false perception of movement or position. Although we think of it as a sensation of revolving or whirling, true vertigo refers to a *sense* or perception of the loss of posture rather than the actual loss itself. Vertigo really is a sense of imbalance, and is difficult to differentiate from dizziness. Medically, dizziness is more a lightheadedness, unsteadiness, faintness, or giddiness rather than a true whirling sensation. For purposes of our discussion, we will regard the two as essentially the same sensation.

Vertigo may be peripheral or central in origin. Peripheral vertigo results from a problem in the end organ or the labyrinth of the inner ear.

Peripheral vertigo is sudden, usually short-lived, and occurs rapidly, frequently with subsequent nausea and vomiting. The vast majority of vertigo attacks are peripheral in origin. Central vertigo results from a problem in the brain itself. Central vertigo tends to be slower in onset and of longer duration. Frequently, other signs of central nervous system abnormalities accompany this kind of vertigo.

Whether central or peripheral, vertigo is characterized by quick, flickerlike movements of the eyes, called nystagmus. These rhythmic, involuntary, back-and-forth movements of the eyes are characteristic of a patient who is suffering acutely from vertigo. If you want to see nystagmus in action, rotate somebody around on a stool for a few times, stop him suddenly, and have him look at your finger, and you will see the nystagmus movements (see Figure 5-19 on page 155). Research on astronauts by recording nystagmus movements electronically has shown that even in a weightless environment, we are all subject to the same stimulus effects on our inner ear with resulting nystagmus and motion sickness.

Weightlessness

In giving talks to pilots, I am frequently asked the question, "What is the effect of weightlessness on vertigo and/or motion sickness?" There has been a considerable amount of research performed on weightlessness. Prior to serious space travel, a 707 was set into a parabolic flight pattern, which produced a zero-G environment and hence weightlessness. However, the research was muddled by the fact that prior to the parabolic curve, G forces had to be exerted upon the experimental subject. Further, the zero-G situation itself lasted for only 15 to 30 seconds. The ultimate experiment was observing the astronauts themselves. This topic was carefully reviewed by a future astronaut-physician, Dr. Geoffrey W. McCarthy, of Westfield, Massachusetts.

Of the several medical problems encountered during space flight, motion sickness has become the chief practical problem for short-duration shuttle missions. Thought to be a "minor problem" in the Gemini and Mercury era, the adverse experiences of early cosmonauts were confirmed on Apollo and especially Skylab flights. Eleven of the 33 Apollo astronauts and seven of the nine Skylab crewmen were affected by motion sickness.

The entire spectrum of signs of motion sickness was observed in these astronauts. Nausea, dizziness, and vomiting affected various Apollo crewmen, and one had persistent dizziness seven days after splashdown. Symptoms were similar in those six Skylab crewmen and were more prevalent after transfer into a more capacious workshop.

For most of us, weightlessness will not pose a problem in the next few years. However, since I do not want us to be misled by early reports that weightlessness does not affect motion sickness, I think it worthy of note here that motion sickness remains as one of the major problems in the weightless state.

Physiology

The physiological cause of motion sickness is stimulation of the inner ear, that devil of a structure that we discussed in our spatial disorientation sections earlier. Stimulation of the inner ear causes all of the central nervous system or somatic or body symptoms that we have described. The more violent the stimulation of the inner ear, the more susceptible our bodies are to motion sickness. Thus, acrobatics, fast turns, high G forces, and inverted flight all subject us to motion sickness.

ANXIETY

There is, of course, a group of people who are motion sick before they leave the ground. Here, the clear-cut cause is anxiety. When you have a passenger who is inexperienced in small-airplane flying, expect motion sickness and prevent it. Prevent it with gentle, skillful piloting. If necessary, advise an antiemetic or antimotion-sickness medication, such as Meclizine, before the flight. (Meclizine is marketed under the trade name Antivert; a 25 mg tablet taken prior to flight may be swallowed or chewed to provide six hours of motion sickness protection.) Lots of reassurance is probably better for your passenger than all of the medication. Keep a motion sickness bag tucked away out of sight in case it is needed. Remember that almost all motion sickness medications detract from mental and/or motor coordination and should not be taken by pilots without prior AME approval.

TREATMENT

Should you feel motion sick, get some cold air on your face, loosen your clothing, use oxygen if

Figure 3-1 demonstrates the effect of positive acceleration, or positive Gs. These are the Gs most commonly experienced. For example, a 60° turn increases our stall factor by placing two Gs on both the airplane and us. As the G effect becomes pronounced, we pool blood. As blood settles toward the feet, vision begins to fade. We gray-out. We still know everything that is happening, but we just can't see the instrument panel or outside the plane adequately. Finally, if we continue, say, a 5-G sustained effort, we black out and thence become unconscious. We can increase our resistance to G forces by tucking our arms in, tucking our chin down, and grunting to force the blood back up to the head. Those of us who have pulled high-G inside loops can well appreciate the protective effect of this maneuver. Fighter pilots wear G suits, illustrated in Figure 3-4, which assist in pushing the blood back up toward the head.

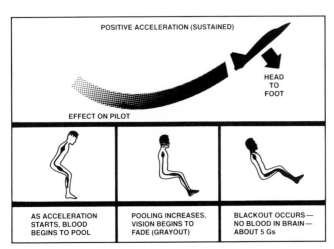

POSITIVE ACCELERATION (SUSTAINED)

HEAD TO FOOT

EFFECT ON PILOT

| AS ACCELERATION STARTS, BLOOD BEGINS TO POOL | POOLING INCREASES, VISION BEGINS TO FADE (GRAYOUT) | BLACKOUT OCCURS— NO BLOOD IN BRAIN— ABOUT 5 Gs |

Figure 3-2 demonstrates the effect of negative acceleration. We appreciate negative acceleration as red-out. Most of our general aviation craft are minimally stressed for negative acceleration or negative Gs. We have all experienced negative acceleration by pushing the controls forward fast and watching our picnic basket drift from the baggage compartment over our head. As we find ourselves lifting out of the seat in a negative-G configuration, blood pools in our head. If we sustain the negative Gs for greater than five seconds, we will red-out. The limit of negative Gs for most of us is three. The end result of moderate negative Gs is usually bleeding into the eyes. Best to avoid! Ask somebody who does outside loops!

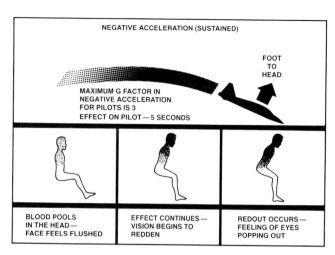

NEGATIVE ACCELERATION (SUSTAINED)

FOOT TO HEAD

MAXIMUM G FACTOR IN NEGATIVE ACCELERATION FOR PILOTS IS 3 EFFECT ON PILOT—5 SECONDS

BLOOD POOLS IN THE HEAD— FACE FEELS FLUSHED

EFFECT CONTINUES— VISION BEGINS TO REDDEN

REDOUT OCCURS— FEELING OF EYES POPPING OUT

you have it, hang onto an outside visual reference point if it is available, and, if not, stay glued to the gyro. Move your eyes and not your head. Remember that even should you become sick, there is nothing wrong with relieving yourself and going back to finishing your flight. One of the best pilots I ever knew, who was consistently a squadron "top gun," was not unknown to return to OPS with his cookies in a bag. Remember, too, that motion sickness is not disqualifying. Should you be subject to motion sickness, perhaps a good discussion with your AME is in order. In any case, your medical supply kit should include motion sickness bags for pilot and passenger.

G FORCES

Accelerative (or G) forces can be important to the general aviation pilot. G refers to gravity. G forces are experienced in 60-degree bank turns (2 Gs), and in many acrobatic maneuvers such as loops (inside or outside). One G is normal weight—what you weigh right now. Two Gs means that you would be pressing into your seat at two times your weight. As you fly your small Cessna Aerobat (see Figure 3-3) around a loop

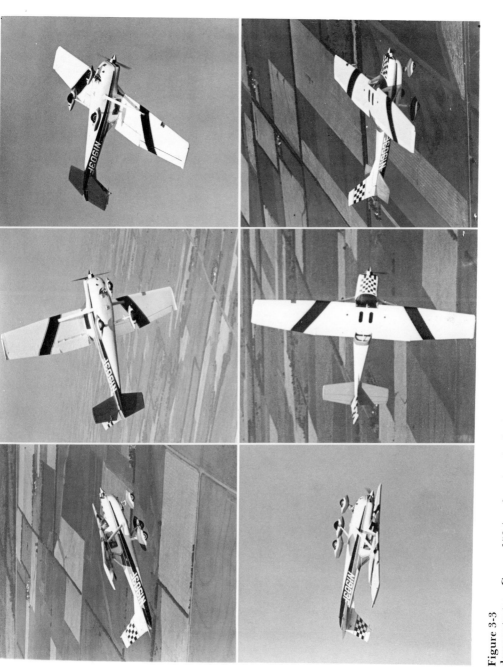

Figure 3-3
demonstrates a Cessna 150 Areobat. Acrobatic airplanes are specifically stressed to handle the higher G forces encountered in acrobatics. They are also equipped with escape mechanisms in order for you to jump out with a parachute if either the airplane or you fail. Acrobatic training is excellent for increasing tolerance to G forces and is worthwhile training for all who fly any aircraft. (Courtesy Cessna Aircraft Corporation)

pattern, you may find that as your G meter moves toward four Gs, you are hard pressed to lift your hand off your lap; it now weighs four times normal. The G force will, of course, hold you in your seat in a positive fashion as you move around the loop. There can be negative Gs, or weightlessness, too. Push your nose forward fast and watch your unattached kneeboard float by your nose, accompanied by the mustard from the picnic lunch in the rear compartment. We can, of course, tolerate many more positive Gs than we can negative Gs (see Figures 3-1 and 3-2).

SYMPTOMS

Without the protection of specially designed transverse seats or G suits (see Figure 3-4), which serve to pump blood from our extremities back up to our brain, there is a limit to the G force that we can tolerate. As we apply positive Gs in a tight turn or loop, blood is not adequately pumped to our head. The eyes, being most sensitive to relative hypoxia, go first. Our vision telescopes in; we begin to see gray; and we lose our instrument panel. If G forces are sustained and/or increased, we black out and lose consciousness.

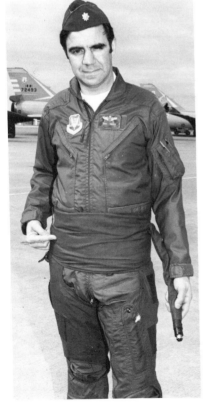

Figure 3-4
demonstrates a G suit which is a zipped-on, constricting, over-the-legs-and-abdomen suit. The pipe on the right is connected to a pressure system in the airplane. As G forces approach two Gs, air is pumped into the G suit, which inflates bladders around the legs and abdomen. These bladders force blood back up into the heart and head, thus increasing the pilot's tolerance to G forces. A G force is nothing more than your weight multiplied by the number of Gs. Thus, if you think of three Gs and you weigh 150 pounds, you will weigh 450 pounds when the G forces are applied. This can be embarrassing if your baggage compartment is certified at 120 pounds and you pull three Gs, leading to a discontinuity in the floor of the airplane. Of more important consequence to the pilot is that, under high G forces, it is virtually impossible for you to lift your hand out of your lap to get at the controls.

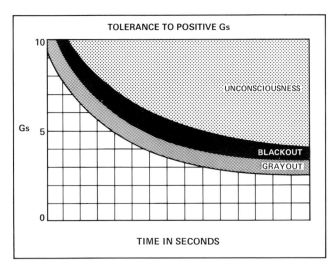

TOLERANCE TO POSITIVE Gs

UNCONSCIOUSNESS

BLACKOUT

GRAYOUT

Gs

TIME IN SECONDS

Figure 3-5
demonstrates our body's tolerance to positive Gs as a function of the *amount* and *time* over which the G forces are applied. It should be obvious that a large number of Gs, say 8, 9, or 10, can be sustained for a short period of time—say one-half to one second. But when you talk about sustained Gs over a longer period of time (say five seconds), most of us are limited to 4 and 4.5 Gs. Those of us active in acrobatics know that we can build our G tolerance with experience and with body position. G-force tolerance is increased by curling up into a fetal position, tucking the head down and grunting. This forces blood into the brain and increases G tolerance. Those of us in combat situations, who routinely fly in an environment of 6 and 7 G forces, are assisted by G suits, as noted in **Figure 3-4.**

Figure 3-6
illustrates the relationship of positive acceleration or G force tolerance to duration. The number of G units as shown on our airplane G meter is represented in the vertical. Note that the amount of time over which we can sustain, say, 10 Gs is only one or two seconds. However, if we look at the 5G level, we find that five to ten seconds can probably be tolerated, although we may enter into the grayout and blackout regions. Three to 4 Gs, over a period of 15 to 20 seconds, is probably a tolerable level for most of us. G forces are tolerated by the younger, better conditioned, and more experienced pilots without difficulty. In fact, many of us flying interceptor planes now are surprised to see that the Air Force no longer requires G suits, since a 4 to 5 G environment is not thought to be particularly dangerous for an experienced pilot. Remember, when we discuss a high-G environment, that *your* tolerance is greater than the tolerance of most of our general aviation airplanes. (See Figure 3-7.)

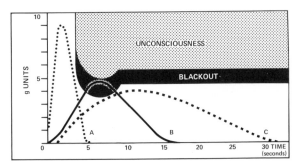

UNCONSCIOUSNESS

BLACKOUT

g UNITS

A   B   C

TIME (seconds)

Figure 3-7
schematically demonstrates our
body's limits to a variety of G forces.
Sustained sources such as turns or
pullouts in an airplane are shown in
#1. The limits, without G suit pro-
tection, vary from individual to individual. In general, we will "gray-
out" at 3 to 4.5 positive Gs. We will
still be conscious, but we will have
difficulty seeing our instrument panel and outside of our airplane. If the
G forces are increased to 5 Gs, we
black out and then become unconscious. In #2, if we are in a dive,
spiral, or spin and want to pull out,
our highest tolerance to 3 Gs is for
about five seconds—assuming our
wings stay on that long. In #3, we
see that we can absorb a high number of Gs for a short interval. Seventeen Gs is perfectly tolerable, but not
for a sustained period of time. In
fact, landings rarely exceed 2 Gs, as
many of us have noted on our airplane's G meters. (Maybe I am not
talking about your landings.) Finally, in #4, even under extreme cata-
pult conditions or rocket launch
conditions, we see that we can tolerate more Gs than can most of our
vehicles. Once again, these are G
forces over short intervals. Bear in
mind, in a nonfighter aircraft (and
that is what most of us fly), our
bodies can take more G forces than
our airplanes.

VARIETY OF G FORCES	
SUSTAINED SOURCES	LIMITS
1. TURNS PULLOUT	GRAYOUT 3 to 4.5 Gs BLACKOUT 4.5 to 5 Gs UNCONSCIOUS 4.5 to 6 Gs
2. DIVES	HIGHEST TOLERANCE 3 Gs for 5 SECONDS
3. LANDINGS	MAXIMUM 17 G RARELY EXCEEDS 2 G
4. CATAPULT	MAXIMUM 12 G RARELY EXCEEDS 2 G

Negative Gs, on the other hand, push blood up to the old squash and we see "red." You can bleed into your eyes and lose consciousness with nega- tive Gs. Thus, blackout for positive Gs and "red- out" for negative Gs are two forces we can impose upon ourselves in a flying environment. We must be familiar with these forces (see Figures 3-5, 3-6 and 3-7).

TREATMENT

How then do we fight off the effects of Gs? In order to sustain positive Gs, we have developed a procedure called the M-1 maneuver. Tuck your arms and legs close to your body; partially close your glottis (voice box); and grunt and strain for all you are worth. This tightens up the abdomi- nal musculature, tenses your muscles, and serves to force blood up to the heart, where it can be pumped back up to the brain. Other than this maneuver, there is little you can do to increase your tolerance. The M-1 maneuver is known to increase tolerance by approximately 1.5 Gs. There is no good method for preventing the effects of negative Gs except to release the Gs.

CHAPTER 4

Physical Causes of Pilot Malfunction

Self-Imposed Destruction

Many stresses, both physiological and emotional, that we place upon ourselves are potentially dangerous to a flier. Physiological stresses range from fatigue, hypoglycemia, alcohol ingestion, dehydration, self-medication, and smoking, to emotional stresses such as anger, frustration, fear, and insecurity. These body stresses are actively increased by noise and vibration associated with reciprocating aircraft, by poor physical fitness in some of us, and by disruptions in the circadian rhythm brought about by flying across time zones. Let's look at these stresses and moderating factors to see more fully how they contribute to difficulties encountered by the pilot.

FATIGUE

Fatigue is characterized by a decrease in flying skill aggravated by physical or emotional stress. Fatigue can be chronic or acute. Chronic fatigue is usually emotional and is frequently produced by boredom or anxiety. Chronic fatigue is frequently not helped by sleeping, but may require medical or psychological assistance. Acute fatigue, in contradistinction to chronic fatigue, is brought on by hard work and can, of course, be reduced by rest. A subacute form of fatigue is task-induced or operational fatigue—fatigue produced by long hours of flying. This type of fatigue is readily treated by a descent, application of wheel blocks, and climbing into a soft cushy bed. Loss of sleep or poor sleeping habits may contribute to both the acute and subacute forms of fatigue.

Symptoms of fatigue are well known to all of us. Their consequences to a flier can be fatal. Skill deteriorates, and flying becomes sloppy. Errors of timing, judgment, and accuracy occur. Forgetfulness follows. The pilot is more irritable and has a loss of sense of humor, and there is an increased tendency for mistakes.

The solution to acute fatigue is obvious. Prevent fatigue by not overstressing or overtaxing your system prior to or during flying. Air Force regulations require a 12-hour crew rest period from the time the engines are shut off until the pilot can report for another briefing. Take a hint from the service with the best safety record. The rationale is clear. We want you, the pilot, to survive another flight. We don't want tiredness and resultant sloppiness to bury you.

HYPOGLYCEMIA

Hypoglycemia, or low blood sugar, produces many of the same symptoms as does fatigue. The low blood sugar is a direct result of either an endocrine disorder such as diabetes, or an improper diet. Since insulin and oral hypoglycemic drugs are disqualifying in fliers, the cause we are most likely to encounter is a poorly balanced diet. The chain of events is frequently predictable. We get up late, are late for our flight, grab a cup of coffee (probably black), file our flight plan, and go. Shortly after we take off, we feel horrible. The symptoms of hypoglycemia have arrived.

Our normal blood sugar of about 100 milligrams percent is being used up and dropping. Symptoms of hypoglycemia, which are similar to those of fatigue, occur: weakness, irritability, poor judgment, and degradation of mental and motor skills. We're saved by the emergency pack in our flight kit, which comes in the form of two beautiful chocolate bars. The chocolate bars are devoured, blood sugar goes sky high, our body compensates by pumping out insulin, which lowers the blood sugar; the blood sugar begins to drop; there are no reserves in our stomach; a new low in blood sugar is achieved; and hypoglycemia is worse than ever. We cannot function well with low blood sugar; we must avoid large shifts up and down in our blood sugar.

The solution to the above dilemma is simple. Eat a well balanced diet. I didn't say a lot—I am not suggesting that we achieve a state of obesity. I am saying that three well-balanced meals each day, which provide adequate vitamins, roughage, and nutrition; and the absence of sugar-laden foods, are the best answer to maintaining homeostasis (an even blood sugar level). A well-balanced diet is the way to avoid hypoglycemia.

The Ideal Diet

A balanced diet should encompass four physiological parameters: 1. basic daily caloric requirements; 2. carbohydrates; 3. protein; and 4. fat. In order to establish a proper diet for yourself, bear in mind the following approximations: 1. Your basic caloric requirements are your pounds in weight multiplied by 10. For example, if you weigh 170 pounds, figure a base of 1,700 calories per day (170 x 10). Of course you have to take into consideration more calories if you are younger, and more calories if you are active. 2. To maintain a carbohydrate balance, a minimum of one gram per pound of body weight is needed. Thus, our 170-pound man would need 170 grams of carbohydrates per day. Since it turns out that each carbohydrate gram contains 4 calories, a total number of 680 calories per day (170 x 4) must be ingested as carbohydrate. 3. Protein requirements are somewhat less and consist of one half gram per pound of body weight per day. Using the same conversion as carbohydrates, you can see that 340 calories must be obtained as protein. 4. Finally, to calculate the amount of dietary fat required, merely subtract the total needed per day of carbohydrates plus protein from the total calories needed per day. Seventeen hundred calories must have taken away from it the 680 carbohydrate calories and the 340 protein calories, which yields the required fat calories of 680 (1,700 minus 680 minus 340). Before you run out to the book store to buy a calorie counter and ideal weight chart, you should know that the society for U.S. Air Force Surgeons has saved you the trouble by publishing ideal weights, a suggested diet, and a neat little calorie counter in their 1979 flight surgeon's checklist. We are including this in Appendix 3 for your use.

The bottom line in an ideal diet is to eat three adequate meals each day. The trick is to maintain a regular and reasonable input without overindulgence at any one point. If we were all success-

ful in doing this while maintaining a modicum
of exercise daily, none of us would be a member
of the "fat club."

Alcohol

Alcohol is related to 60 percent of automobile
accidents. Similarly, many general aviation accidents are alcohol-related. It behooves us all to
understand something about the problem of
alcohol and flying. The real problem is that
alcohol affects flying more than it does driving.
The two after-work cocktails with which we
safely drove home are made more powerful by
hypoxia when we fly. What may be a safe level at
sea level is accelerated to a disruptive, degrading
level at altitude, and subsequent disaster. Because
flying is a more finely honed skill than driving,
what we can get away with on the ground, we
can't in the air. Furthermore, alcohol itself
produces nystagmus; nystagmus is characteristic
of vertigo and motion sickness.

Following alcohol ingestion, peak blood levels
are found in one hour. The amount of alcohol in
the blood is a determining factor as to how
"drunk" we get. In order to relate alcoholic
beverages to real-life situations, a convenient
chart and nomogram is provided in Appendix 4,
which shows you how much alcohol is present in
varying amounts of varying beverages. To trans-
late shots of alcohol into blood levels (see Figure
4-1), bear in mind that there is a slight variation
with the weight of the flier and his ability to
metabolize alcohol. The metabolism of common
drinks and its relation to input is explained in
Figure 4-2. See Appendix 4 for clinical status
related to blood alcohol levels. Suffice it to say

Figure 4-1 demonstrates blood alcohol levels following a given dose of alcohol. Bear is mind that 50 mg%, or the blood level achieved after one ounce of alcohol is consumed, is legally considered enough for drunk driving in most states. Of course, this level is potentiated by hypoxia in the flying environment. You can readily understand how only a small number of drinks will provide a blood alcohol level that in an airplane can prove disastrous.

APPROXIMATE BLOOD ALCOHOL LEVELS FOLLOWING A DOSE OF ALCOHOL

Below 0.05% (50 mg%)	1
0.05% (50 mg%)–0.10% (100 mg%)	2
0.10% (100 mg%)–0.15% (150 mg%)	4
0.15% (150 mg%)–0.20% (200 mg%)	6
0.20% (200 mg%)–0.25% (250 mg%)	8
0.25% (250 mg%)–0.30% (300 mg%)	10
0.30% (300 mg%)–0.40% (400 mg%)	12

BLOOD ALCOHOL LEVEL[a]	AMOUNT INGESTED[b]
Below 0.50% (50 mg%)	1
0.05%–0.10% (50-100 mg%)	2

[a]Maximum absorption levels in minimum time; figures based on average body weight of 70 kg.

[b]For purposes of estimation, 1 bottle of beer (12 oz.) equals 1 oz. of distilled spirit (80–90 proof).

that two ounces of 87-proof whiskey produces a blood alcohol level of 50 milligrams percent; the same alcohol level is achieved with two 12-ounce cans of beer. This level interferes with flying. (About 10 percent of fatal accidents in 1978 were attributed to alcohol, according to NTSB data, which employ 50 milligrams percent or over as a significant level.) How long does it take to clear this alcohol? It has been estimated that 10 to 15 milligrams percent per hour or about one ounce or shot per three hours is metabolized. Therefore, you can plan on well over four to five hours before your blood alcohol level approaches normal. The question then becomes, Shall I fly after I know there is no alcohol left in my blood?

Unfortunately, the effects of alcohol are felt long after the blood level achieves a zero mark. The FAA has taken the position "eight hours from bottle to throttle." The Air Force, realizing the length of time it takes for the body to overcome the effects of alcohol, has taken a position of 24 hours from drinking to flying. The reason for the more stringent service regulation is that alcohol is a histotoxic drug and serves to block oxygen uptake in the tissues. This results, then, in hypoxic and/or hypoglycemia symptoms, even though the alcohol has been metabolized from the body. This author published early research showing that alcohol robbed the body of necessary dream time, thus accounting for a feeling of fatigue even after eight hours of sleep. The point should be quite clear. Drinking and flying do not go together. An FAA brochure called *Alcohol and Flying Don't Mix* (Aviation Medical Education Series #5) sums it all up in its final warning:

If you're going to sip, delay the trip.

There is a disturbing absence of valid research in the civilian population regarding the influence of alcohol in nonfatal accidents. The absence of a clear association between alcohol and *nonfatal* accidents speaks more for the lack of documentation than it does for the lack of alcohol in many of these pilots. Let us not be misled by statistics that can be skewed to make the point of the investigator. Those of us familiar with pilots, many of whom are involved in repeated small episodes, know all too well that a small amount of alcohol produces disturbing results in the pilot.

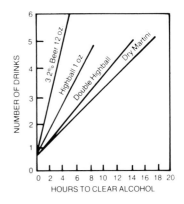

APPROXIMATE TIME REQUIRED FOR ELIMINATION OF ALCOHOL FROM VARIOUS KINDS OF DRINKS

Figure 4-2

demonstrates the time required to eliminate alcohol from various kinds of drinks. Look at the number of drinks on the vertical as we increase to six and extend out the number of hours necessary to clear this alcohol. If you take a martini, for example, you can see that 16 hours plus are needed to clear the alcohol from your blood. Thus, the eight-hour "bottle-to-throttle" rule imposed by the FAA is surely a minimum. You are far safer to accept the Air Force recommendation of 24 hours "bottle-to-throttle" to make certain all alcohol has been removed from the body. The effects of alcohol are not limited to the direct blood-level effect, but extend beyond the time of all alcohol removed from the body. Indirect effects may include fatigue, hypoglycemia, and dehydration.

Dehydration

Dehydration must be avoided, especially by pilots. Dehydration leads to degradation of both motor and mental performance by mimicking many of the same symptoms present with hypoglycemia, fatigue, and alcohol ingestion. Dehydration leads to irritability, a general feeling of discomfort, sleepiness, and dizziness. In its more extreme state, headache and then physiological collapse progress. How then can we avoid dehydration?

Dehydration can be avoided by ingesting adequate amounts of water at regular intervals and by avoiding drugs that produce dehydration. Increased heat and labor increase the need for water. The solution to maintaining an adequate water level is to drink an adequate amount of water before you leave and carry enough water on board so that dehydration or drying out of the body will never become a problem for you. Drugs that lead to dehydration usually produce their effect by increasing water loss in the urine. Some medications, such as diuretics, which are used to treat hypertension, are disqualifying in pilots. The two most common drugs that produce dehydration in pilots are caffeine and alcohol.

Both caffeine and alcohol act to increase water loss by increasing urination (diuresis). These drugs act in an identical fashion. Caffeine and alcohol suppress antidiuretic hormone (ADH) secretion from the pituitary gland. ADH presence is needed to reabsorb water filtered from the blood through the kidneys. When antidiuretic hormone is suppressed, water loss through the kidneys is increased because reabsorption is decreased. This results in an increased amount of urine and a decreased amount of water available within the body. It seems parodoxical that the beers some people drink on a hot sunny day in fact produce the opposite effect from what is desired; they do not adequately replace body water. The effects of dehydration from both alcohol and caffeine are, of course, felt long after the drug has departed the body. Hence the warning—if you know you are

exposed to drugs that dehydrate, keep an adequate water load on board (body and ship) to
compensate for the induced water loss.

Self-Medication

You should not be flying while taking medication. Medication does not refer necessarily to a
prescription, but applies to many over-the-
counter preparations as well. Even the most innocent of medications, such as aspirin and cold
remedies, can seriously impair your ability to fly,
withstand motion sickness, and/or survive an
accident. The most important point to remember
is to consult your AME prior to taking any
medication before flying.

Bear in mind that almost all pharmaceuticals
taken on a chronic basis are disqualifying for
flying unless you have a waiver for flying with
them. Bear in mind also that you have "the final
responsibility" in determining your ability to fly
(see Chapter 1). Taking medication implies that
you are ill; if you are ill, you don't belong in the
air.

There are many reasons why the most innocent
of illnesses is activated in the air. Take the
common cold, for example. Not life threaten-
ing—at least while you're on the ground. The
excess swelling of the mucous membranes of the
nose, sinuses, and ears compromises the ability of
the sinuses and the ears to equalize pressure. As
we begin to descend, should the passage to the ear
and/or sinus not open, severe pain, sometimes
bleeding, and sometimes incredible vertigo result.
Thus, the most innocent of infirmities can result
in a tragedy. On the back side of the equation is
the combined cold remedy that contains an
antihistamine and an adrenaline compound. The

adrenaline peps us up and makes us feel pretty good. We extend ourselves beyond our physical ability and run into trouble, say, by shooting an IFR approach; if the adrenaline doesn't get us, the antihistamine will. Side effects of antihistamines include drowsiness and disorientation, both of which are potentiated by hypoxia. There just is no profit in self-medication; there is no profit in flying when you are ill.

Problems of medication in flying are not confined to those drugs taken for simple illnesses. Occasionally even the most innocent medications can produce side effects, which in the pilot lead to an accident. For example, laxatives taken for constipation can become potassium depleters. With lack of potassium, confusion, a tendency for heat irritability, and weakness follow. On the other side of the coin, should the laxative not be successful, impacted feces in the bowels create trapped gas, as discussed in Chapter 2; the result of what would be an innocent problem on the ground is catastrophic as the bowels rupture at altitude. Many medications, such as diet pills, have side effects hardly noticed on the ground but potentiated in the air. False confidence because of a "high" feeling as well as disorientation and easy incapacitation, with vertigo-producing disorientation, are readily brought on in fliers taking diet pills. We could go on and on. The point should be quite clear. Even patent medications or over-the-counter preparations have no business in your system while you are in the air.

This subject could be more readily understood if the effects of medications were predictable in each individual. Unfortunately, drug effects frequently extend above and beyond their desired purpose and administration. Reactions to drugs extend from simple idiosyncratic reactions, such as a rash, to a full-blown anaphylactic shock with

COMMON DRUG SIDE EFFECTS

1.	Cold preparations	Drowsiness
		Incoordination
		Vertigo
		Motion sickness
2.	Aspirin	Increased bleeding
3.	Cathartics	Dehydration
		Confusion
		Heart irritability
4.	Antidiarrheals	Incoordination
		Confusion
5.	Tranquilizers	Reduced alertness
		Incoordination
6.	Painkillers	Decreased mental alertness
		Decreased coordination
7.	Antibiotics	Diarrhea
		Anaphylactic collapse
8.	Immunizations	Allow 24 hours to avoid fever, fatigue, and incoordination

Figure 4-3.
Many common over-the-counter and prescribed drugs can have serious side effects even while you're on the ground. In the air, the danger is even greater.

subsequent incapacitation and death (see Figure 4-3). Adverse reactions such as nausea, vomiting, tremors, incoordination, and rigidity of muscles can all occur from such innocent medications as antimotion-sickness drugs (e.g., Meclizine). Effects of drugs are frequently activated by the flier's environment, which includes decreased pressure, hypoxia, and sometimes increased G forces in steep banks, sudden dives, or thunderstorms. Occasionally, the effect of a drug on another medication already in the system potentiates that second medication's effect. For example, systemic or body uptake from nose sprays can lead to severe reactions in patients with blood-pressure problems and in patients taking antidepressants. So your concern need not be limited to yourself but also must extend to your passengers. Medicine and flying do not mix unless they are approved by your AME.

Self-medication may be a fact of life. It is naive

for doctors to expect that a significant portion of the American population do not medicate themselves, and that an even greater percentage are not taking medicine prescribed by physicians other than their flight medical examiner. That doesn't mean that I advocate flying while medicated. I don't. But the sagest advice that I can give you, *should* you decide to bend the regulation (bending is illegal), is to be honest with yourself. If you don't know the effect of medication on your flying, you are a fool to try it for the first time. The military has a policy of providing pilots who are going on long tours of duty with certain stimulants and certain depressants. But no pilot can be issued such medication without a ground trial of the medication and a questionnaire that has evaluated various facets of performance and feelings. Learn from the experience of those who are in the business. Medicine and flying do not mix, and medicine without a trial belongs *nowhere* in flying.

Smoking

I once had an instructor whose main beef with smokers was that the residue in the cockpit plugged up the capillary tubes in his vertical-speed indicator. My gripe with smokers is that the residue carbon monoxide left in their lungs makes hypoxia an inevitable sequela to their flying. It has been estimated that three cigarettes a day or one cigar a day places us, physiologically, at 8,000 feet. The smoker is well advised to start using oxygen above 5,000 feet. Let's look at some of the reasons cigarette smoking produces such physiologically degrading carbon monoxide levels.

It is true that carbon monoxide can leak into our cockpit through heat vent flow over a leaking muffler system. This is the reason why so many of us have carbon monoxide detecting buttons hanging in our small planes. With the number of smokers in this country, far and away the chief cause of carbon monoxide poisoning is not a defective heating system but rather the self-pollution we bring upon ourselves. Carbon monoxide makes up somewhere under five percent of the cigarette smoke that we inhale. Carbon monoxide is taken into the lungs and attracted to the red blood cell hemoglobin 200 times more actively than is oxygen. The affinity of carbon monoxide for hemoglobin is incredible; hemoglobin gobbles carbon monoxide. The carbon monoxide stays put. Carbon monoxide does not diffuse into the tissues, but rather takes the hemoglobin out of circulation so that it is not available for oxygen carrying. Thus the flier or passenger is anemic before he begins his flight. Symptoms of carbon monoxide poisoning are well delineated in Appendix 6. As a smoker, you would not think of yourself as carbon monoxide poisoned. But you are, as soon as you leave the ground. The decreased oxygen available to your tissues has decreased your night vision by 20 percent and increased your body's heat production by over 10 percent. The pack-and-a-half-a-day cigarette smoker has 10 percent of his hemoglobin bound up by carbon monoxide, which at a service ceiling of 10,000 feet has placed him physiologically at 15,000 feet during the day and even higher at night. You do not clear your body of its carbon monoxide level by not having a cigarette for eight hours prior to flight. Carbon monoxide is stuck to those red blood cells for days and weeks. So you're stuck to an oxygen bottle above 5,000 feet. Use it. Use it at all altitudes at night. If you insist on destroying yourself by smoking, at least carry oxygen!

Fear of Flying

I recall all too vividly a 3,000-hour fighter pilot coming into my office one day and saying, "Doc, I'm just afraid to fly at night." Do you find this bewildering? I don't. It's the unusual experienced pilot who has not had second thoughts about jumping into the sky on certain days. I am not confining my observations to a pilot before his first solo, before his instrument check ride, before his first flight with his family, or while descending at 10,000 feet a minute in a thunderstorm. I am talking about any of us with a modicum of experience who has an inner voice that suddenly says, "Stay the hell out of the sky."

The most important treatment for this sensation is its recognition. I have never heard of a nut who knew he was nuts. The recognition that "something is wrong" is healthy and normal. There are times when the best way to fly is to make a 180 and walk away from the airplane. Given a normal day with a little bit of experience under your belt and a sensation that "everything ain't right"—that is the time to walk. Come back for another try.

The more distressing fear of flying situations are those in which the pilot is upset, is unafraid, and jumps into the left seat anyhow. As you know, the neuropsychiatric portion of the FAA history and exam is important. Everything from minor mental disorders to psychoses are disqualifying. No, we are not talking about somebody who has been hospitalized with a mental disorder, or who had a predisposition to shoot up or drink himself into a stupor. We are talking about all of us—normal everyday flying folk who are subject to the impacts of the world around us. We don't belong in the seat flying after a fight with our wife, after we have just been fired from our job, or if we are just plain worried, about anything. The emotional state in the cockpit has to be one of tranquillity. Not that some apprehension under abnormal flying conditions can't be healthy. In fact, the increased pulse and respiration associated with adrenaline output under stressful situations can actually make us more finely tuned to pull off, say, a "to bare minimum" IFR approach. But anxiety, upset, frustration or depression don't belong in your head while you are flying. If you are upset, do something else.

While we are on the subject of being upset, think about your passenger. I have been in eight-G breaks, dive-bomb runs heading toward the earth at 45 degrees indicating 500 knots, in five-G loops, and rudder-rolling the airplane 10 times in succession, but I have never been so scared as I was on my own first flight. Have some compassion for your passenger, who may not have your experience. Demonstrations of stalls, spirals, chandelles, lazy eights, or whatever else you happen to think represents "skilled flying," have no place on your passenger's maiden voyage itinerary. Concentrate on preflighting your passenger so that he is convinced of the inherent safety of those incredible flying machines. Let him know what is going to happen before it happens. Stick to 20-degree banks, smooth air, and a single landing with no bounces. You want that passenger back to fly with you again and perhaps to take lessons himself. You should always have a motion-sickness bag available (but out of sight). Don't hesitate to give an apprehensive passenger an antimotion-sickness drug such as Meclizine. Make sure that a pregnant passenger has checked with her obstetrician regarding the advisability of flying above 2,000 or 3,000 feet. Give some thought as to whether or not your passenger may have any cardiac or pulmonary problems. Remember that *you* are responsible for the health and safety of your passengers. Surely you would not wish to feel responsible for their discomfort in return for your trying to give them a good time.

Fearing weather is different from respecting weather. We should do our best to anticipate weather conditions. This can frequently be accomplished by observing the TV weather forecast the day of or before flight and then getting the latest update from the flight service station. But losing sleep and worrying about what is going to happen has never saved anybody. Respecting the weather, preparing for it, and avoiding conditions in which it's not advisable to fly are the only ways to keep a plane from biting.

An emotionally stable state and a feeling of relaxation, so that everything is just right, leads to better flying. I am not saying that we should be so relaxed that we are lax. I am saying that when we are scared, nervous, or when we lack self-discipline we are not going to do our best in a ticklish situation. Not that a little apprehension doesn't sometimes help. Our sympathetic response, which speeds up our heart and pumps adrenaline through our system, alerts us to the "flight from fright" readiness. But it is a very different situation from being aroused at the time of the emergency to work more efficiently and being nervous about it from the start so that we are all expended when the moment of truth arrives.

An example of a tough place to keep cool is in a thunderstorm. Even the most careful of pilots—given enough time in the air—is bound to mix it up with a thunderstorm. Believe me, it is an experience. It is tough to hang onto your gauges; it is tough to hang onto your plane. You are tempted to make a 180. But sometimes it is a lot harder to make a turn with 10,000 fpm up- and downdrafts, and an instrument panel that just keeps jiggling, than it is to just try and hold your wings level and say a prayer. Crank up the light so that you are not flash blinded, keep the wings level, and hang on to your pants. If your airplane doesn't come apart, you'll make it.

The psychology of flying need not be complex. Robert N. Buck, in his book, *Weather Flying,* while discussing the psychology of weather flying summed it up in one word: self-discipline. This really says it all. To be scared or white-knuckled under adverse conditions is only normal. In fact, some of the fright-in-flight stimulation serves to move us physically into a more efficacious position to tackle a serious problem. Control of one's mind is the cornerstone of good flying. Self-discipline is really nothing more than maturity. Your second chances are limited in flying. So condition yourself to think clearly and always to exhibit self-control. Many of us have heard the story over and over of the VFR-rated pilot who flew into IFR conditions, was assisted by the ground controllers and followed meticulously on a radarscope while he performed beautifully. Then the pilot was faced with one final emergency as his gas ran low. He panicked and spun in. He could have and should have made it. The only difference between the winner and the loser is that one maintains his confidence and cool, and the other blows it. Think positively. You can do it if you want to do it and if you know you can do it.

Noise and Vibration

Noise and vibration fatigue pilots and passengers alike. They interfere with communication

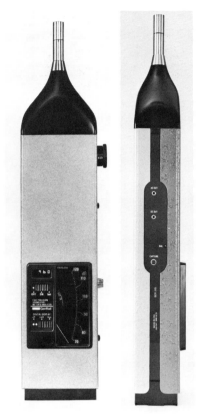

Figure 4-4.
Front and side view of progressive sound level meter used to determine the decibels or intensity of sound on an aircraft ramp or in the cockpit. (Courtesy GenRad, Inc.)

during and sometimes after flight, and lead to permanent hearing disabilities. It has long been known that excess vibration, whether on the back of a jackhammer or in the cockpit of a reciprocating aircraft, leads to excessive fatigue and many other somatic, or body, problems (e.g., hypertension). There is not too much we can do to eliminate the vibration in flying, but we surely can do something about the noise.

Only recently have we recognized the problems associated with long-term noise exposure. We know that workers employed in industry under noisy conditions for many years frequently end up deaf. We know that artillerymen and marksmen exposed to short but high-intensity noise frequently end up deaf. Legislation was first introduced in 1969 as the Walsh-Healey Act and finalized in 1971 as the Occupational Safety and Health Act (OSHA)—this legislation serves to limit the maximum noise exposure Americans may sustain under a variety of conditions. Let's look at how this noise is measured, how much is present in the flying environment, and what we can do to protect ourselves from noise-induced hearing loss.

The intensity of noise is a function of the sound pressure level, which is measured in decibels (dB), usually by a sound level meter (see Figure 4-4). The intensity in decibels of the noise can be measured over a host of frequencies, but the most important frequencies range from 300 to 4,800 Hertz, or cycles per second. For the purpose of our discussion the broad-band noise covering this large frequency range is termed "white noise." We must consider the damage sustained by our ears as a function of the intensity of this white noise over a period of time. The OSHA Act has set certain limits of noise exposure that are considered safe (see Figure 4-5). When either the

1910.95—OCCUPATIONAL NOISE EXPOSURE

(a) Protection against the effects of noise exposure shall be provided when the sound levels exceed those shown in Table G-16 when measured on the A scale of a standard sound level meter at slow response. When noise levels are determined by octave band analysis, the equivalent A-weighted sound level may be determined as follows:

(b)
(1) When employees are subjected to sound exceeding those listed in Table G-16, feasible administration or engineering controls shall be utilized. If such controls fail to reduce sound levels within the levels of Table G-16, personal protection equipment shall be provided and used to reduce sound levels within the levels of the table.

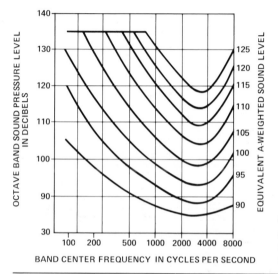

BAND CENTER FREQUENCY IN CYCLES PER SECOND

TABLE G–16—PERMISSIBLE NOISE EXPOSURES

Duration per day, hours	Sound level dBA slow response
8	90
6	92
4	95
3	97
2	100
1½	102
1	105
½	110
¼ or less	115

When the daily noise exposure is composed of two or more periods of noise exposure of different levels, their combined effect should be considered, rather than the individual effect of each.

intensity and/or the time noted is exceeded, noise-induced hearing loss can result (see Figure 4-6).

It is well known that many small private airplanes have potentially damaging noise levels exceeding 95 dB. Jets, especially in afterburner, produce even higher levels of sound intensity, sometimes exceeding 115–120 dB. There are three methods that can be employed in reducing exposure to noise: isolate the noise, insulate the noise, protect the pilot. It is obvious that the pilot's only alternative is to insulate himself. Insulation or self-protection can be accomplished

Figure 4-5
is an extract from the OSHA regulations regarding noise exposure. All pilots should be well aware of the damage risk criteria to the human ear, since airport ramps are always noisy. In particular, glance at Table G-16 and bear in mind that most general aviation craft—especially older craft—exceed 95 dB to 100 dB in noise intensity. Since we know our exposure to this noise is likely to be longer than the permissible noise exposure times, we should wear ear protection in light aircraft.

EAR NOSE AND THROAT ASSOCIATES, INC.

RICHARD B. YULES, M.D.
MARSHALL J. ZAMANSKY, M.D.
STEPHEN R. KURLAND, M.D.

PLEASANT MEDICAL CENTER NORTH
475 PLEASANT STREET
WORCESTER, MASS. 01609
AREA CODE 617
791-6305

MEDICAL ARTS BUILDING
100 SOUTH STREET
SOUTHBRIDGE, MASS. 01550
AREA CODE 617
765-5461

HEAD AND NECK SURGERY
OTOLOGY
BRONCHOESOPHAGOSCOPY

FACIAL PLASTIC SURGERY
OTONEUROLOGY
MAXILLO-FACIAL SURGERY

AUDIOMETRIC REPORT

NAME _____ AGE _____ DATE _____ 19 ____

EAR SX _____ TESTER _____ INSTRUMENT 6S-1702

PREOP _____ POSTOP _____ TEST VALIDITY:G ____ F ____ P ____

PURE TONE AUDIOGRAM

Weber
L   R

FREQUENCY IN CYCLES PER SECOND

Hearing Threshold Level in dB (Ansi, 1969)

CRITICAL SPEECH AREA

AMA % HEARING LOSS: R ____ L ____ BINAURAL ____

COMMENTS:

Bilateral Tinnitus approaches narrow band

noise centered around 6000 Hz at a 15 db sensation

level.

48-2M-LAIT-2/79C

MLV ____ TAPE ____

SPEECH RECEPTION THRESHOLD

	dB	MASK	SAT	BONE
R	5			
L	10			
SF				

DISCRIMINATION (LIST _____)

	%	LEVEL	MASK
R	72	50	
L	72	50	
BI			
SF			

TONE DECAY

Hz			
R			
L			

SISI

Hz			
R			
L			

STENGER: POS _____ NEG _____

BEKESY: _____

ABLB: _____

MASKING LEVEL IN NON-TEST EAR

	AIR	BONE	
R			NBN ____
L			BBN ____

	AIR	MASK	BONE	MASK
R		Δ	>	▶
L	x	□	<	◀

Figure 4-6

is an audiogram of a pilot with a noise-induced hearing loss. Note the marked loss of hearing in the 4,000 to 6,000 hertz, or cycles, per second, range with a rebound of some hearing at 8,000 hertz. This curve with a notch in the 4,000- to 6,000-hertz range is characteristic of trauma or noise-induced hearing loss. The hearing loss is irreversible and is assisted not at all by amplification.

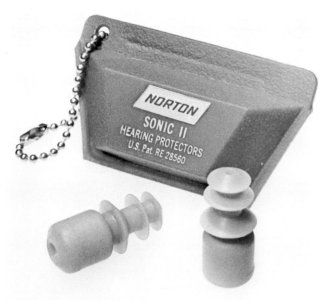

Figure 4-7

shows a typical earplug. Earplugs should be employed in cases where airplanes are not equipped to accept headsets and/or where headsets are not available or affordable. Earplugs offer almost the same protection as earmuffs, but with less comfort. A good method for inserting an earplug is to grasp the ear around the back of the head with the opposite hand, thus stretching out the ear canal and allowing for the easy insertion of the earplug. Keep the earplugs clean.

with either earplugs or earmuffs. Earplugs (see Figures 4-7, 4-8 and 4-9) serve to reduce the noise level in the cockpit. Surprisingly enough, they also make speech discrimination from the overhead speaker more intelligible. It is almost a contradiction to expect to hear better by hearing less, but this is what happens. Lower the noise level by wearing earplugs in a noisy environment, and you will actually hear better. If you find the earplugs uncomfortable or impractical, the next step is to purchase earmuffs with a phone inserted (see Figure 4-10). Here you have the best of both worlds. Clear headphone reception is combined with protection from aircraft noise using a soundproof muff. As can be seen in Figure 4-11, the decrease of noise to the ear with either a plug or a muff is marked. In general, you can obtain a 30 dB decrement in noise levels in the speech frequencies with the use of appropriate ear

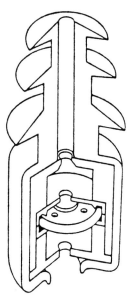

Figure 4-8
shows a cutaway view of the valve of the Sonic II ear protector.
(Courtesy Norton Company)

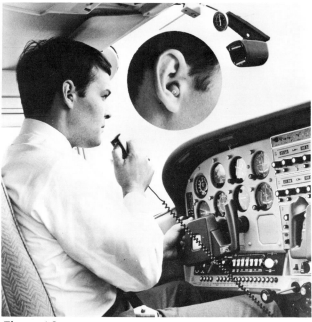

Figure 4-9
illustrates an ear protector in the pilot's ear during flight. This ear protector is comfortable and offers sufficient protection against ambient noise levels in general aviation aircraft. The same ear protector will suffice as protection on the ramp.
(Courtesy Norton Company)

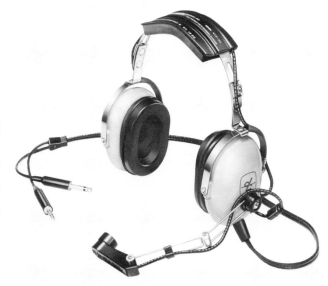

Figure 4-10
demonstrates an ideal combination of communication and protection of our ears from aircraft noise. By allowing us to hear with a headset imbedded in noise-protective earmuffs, we combine the best of both worlds. We maintain a quiet environment while placing the source of communication close to our heads. At the same time, the microphone gives us a hands-off capability for controlling the airplane.
(Courtesy David Clark Company)

114

ATTENUATION DATA

ATTENUATION IN DECIBELS (dB)	FREQUENCY IN HERTZ (Hz)
Frequency (Hz)	Model H10-30
125	17
*Std. Dev.	2.2
250	25
Std. Dev.	3.1
500	33
Std. Dev.	3.8
1000	35
Std. Dev.	1.8
12000	38
Std. Dev.	3.3
3000	46
Std. Dev.	3.9
4000	46
Std. Dev.	4.9
6000	42
Std. Dev.	3.6
8000	38
Std. Dev.	4.1

*Standard Deviation

Figure 4-11 demonstrates headset features and attenuation data for a typical headset. This decrement of noise of roughly 30 dB–40 dB (decibels) is adequate to make even a noisy private airplane nondamaging to the human ear. Ear protection is strongly recommended for all civil aviation pilots.
(Courtesy David Clark Company)

protection. This brings the sound level reaching your ear down to a more than safe level and makes flying a pleasure instead of a hazard. Why not have a set of ear protectors for your passenger, too?

Fitness and Age

Physical fitness is as important to flying as it is to daily life. To file a good flight plan, preflight the airplane well, and let yourself, a "physical wreck," jump into the pilot's seat doesn't make good sense. The bottom line in safe flying is the guy pushing the buttons. Self-respect and concern for yourself are as important in being a good pilot as the preflight inspection, flight plan, and the plane itself.

What about the effect of age on pilot performance? Appropriate tests for pilot proficiency are not employed. We do, however, have an age distribution based on FAA computer printouts of the number of pilots in any age group and their accident rates. The findings speak well for the old hats. A curve can be drawn showing a low accident rate in the young group and a low accident rate in the older pilots. Contrary to statistics accumulated for automobile drivers, the under-20 fliers tend to have fatal accidents in airplanes half as often as would be expected. The 20-to-30 age group also does well. It is middle-of-the-roaders, between 35 and 40, who have the worst record. But as we get to the old hats, the statistics improve progressively. Pilots in their early 50s do better than the younger, middle-aged pilots and the 55-to-60 age group does even better. The point for the moms and dads, grandmas and grandpas is not to give up flying because the years are flitting by. There is no evidence suggesting that growing older decreases your ability to pilot an aircraft. If anything, among the old hats, the maturity of age, the decisions engendered by weathered judgment, and the lessened desire to take chances all serve to more than compensate for the lack of physical stamina, poor eyesight, poor hearing, and weaker hearts we all are bound to develop.

In 1959, the FAA instituted an "age-60 rule," which prohibits an individual from serving as a pilot in an air carrier and certain other flight operations after reaching his or her 60th birthday. This rule has been challenged in the courts repeatedly, but the FAA has consistently won favorable decisions. On December 5, 1979, a challenge, originally introduced into the U.S. House of Representatives, that would have effectively raised the age limit to 61½ years was amended, so that current legislation entering 1981 leaves the age-60 rule unaltered. As of the date of this writing, no action has taken place in the U.S. Senate.

Circadian Rhythm

Circadian rhythm describes the cycles of activity in our bodies; the cycles wax and wane over every 24 hours or so. The word *circadian* means "around a day" and was originally used by Dr. Franz Halberg. Dr. Halberg is the founding father of chronobiology research, which delves into the circadian rhythms. The value of circadian rhythm to pilots is obvious. If there are certain periods of the day when we are more effective or efficient, these are the periods during which we should strive to fly. It therefore merits a look at chronobiology so that we may extract those facets that we may apply to our flying activities.

There are a multitude of biological functions that wax and wane over time. Very few of the measures of our body, which we routinely take in physical and laboratory studies, are constant. For example, our hematocrit, or our concentration of red blood cells, will tend to be higher during the morning, but will be some five percent lower during our mid-sleeping hours. Our waking temperatures are usually lower than our midday temperatures. Ovulating women tend to have a higher temperature during their peak ovulation period. Blood sugars tend to be low in the morning and higher after we have eaten. All of these factors are not true for some segments of the population—in our "night owls" whose circadian rhythm is almost reversed. Furthermore, physicians are coming to realize that circadian rhythms may be exploited in maximizing patient therapy results. We have found, for example, that an anti-cancer drug (Doxorubicin) when given early in the morning is metabolized very differently from the same dose when given one-half day later. Similar experiments have been performed on mice on anti-cancer drugs and have resulted in over a 50 percent cure when given, say, early in the morning, but only a 15 percent cure when given in mid to late morning. We have extended these observations in the treatment of hypertensive patients, where we have found that a diuretic is much more effective when given early in the morning than when given 12 hours later in the evening. Let's extend some of these types of data to the treatment of jet lag in fliers.

The Army is currently experimenting with using chronobiology to make its fighting troops more effective when they land on foreign soil. Their initial experiments were based on several observations: 1. methylated xanthines such as are found in tea and coffee tend to advance the body clock, depending on when they are ingested; 2. food initiates the circadian rhythm cycle, especially when taken on an empty stomach; 3. protein initiates synthesis of chemicals (catecholamines), which initiate active phases of the circadian rhythm; and 4. carbohydrates tend to favor sugar production, which is higher during sleep or emotional states. Using these four pieces of information, Army scientists organized an experiment with 90 men.

The men departed at noon, Eastern Standard Time, for Germany. Prior to takeoff, they had a small breakfast and decaffeinated coffee. Following departure, they were told to advance their watches six hours to the local German time. A small high-protein lunch was fed to them as a "supper," and they were put to bed before six

P.M., their local time. Remember, it is now midnight in Germany. After five hours, they were awakened to a high-protein breakfast of steak and eggs with a lot of nice black coffee. Their German-reading watches now read early in the morning (five A.M.). They then landed in Germany, and a multitude of biologic evaluations were carried out for the next several days. These findings were compared with those of an additional 90 men transported with no special treatment. The results all suggest that the circadian rhythm can be modified to markedly diminish jet lag.

Much more work needs to be done on the circadian rhythm. Evolving studies tend to help us in establishing a pattern that will be helpful in making us alert pilots—both mentally and physically. Get a good eight-hour rest prior to departure. Use a limited amount of coffee for breakfast, and stick with a high-protein and low-carbohydrate meal prior to flight. All of these maneuvers will serve to keep your circadian rhythm in the best possible shape for good pilotage.

Lest our chronobiology, or circadian rhythm comments, be confused with biorhythm, let us devote one paragraph to the biorhythm myth. Biorhythm has been ballyhooed as "not science fiction, but medical fact." Co-discovered by a psychologist, Hermann Swoboda, and an otolaryngologist, Wilhelm Fliess, both of whom were contemporaries of Sigmund Freud, biorhythm is promoted as a cycle wherein everyone's physical, emotional, and intellectual life is governed by three cycles. The cycles begin at birth. Physical well-being falls and rises over a 23-day cycle, emotional highs and lows flow over a 28-day cycle, and intellectual ups and downs range over a 33-day cycle. There has been a host of material produced on biorhythm, much of which was pushed by George Thommen. Thommen claimed that a study of 300 deaths demonstrated that 65 percent of the deaths occurred on those few days in the year (15 percent) critical for the individuals based on the above odd-day cycles. A National Institute of Health researcher, Dr. Manning Feinlib, has recently torpedoed these data in researching 960 deaths; he found no association between the death days and the so-called critical days. Although this is not a proper forum for disputing the biorhythm theory, it suffices to say that physicians are not convinced of its merits. Neither the FAA nor the military flight surgeons have any recommendations regarding its acceptance. Biorhythm is not to be confused with circadian rhythm, which appears to have a basis in scientific fact and documentation.

The physiological or metabolic clock produces the circadian rhythm peculiar to each of us. During the day we are "up for it;" during the night we are in a relaxed state, dreaming, and with our body functions depressed. Anytime we fly beyond our local time zone, we are subject to an imposed stress on our body because we try to live outside of our established circadian rhythm. The most obvious example is a jet jaunt across the ocean to a foreign country, perhaps arriving at a local time not too different from the time at the trip's inauguration. Thus the term "jet lag." If we start off where we began we're bound to end up fatigued, perhaps with a bowel upset, and surely behind the eight ball when we climb back into the plane to resume our activities.

How, then, do we cope with time changes? The most important principle is to over-rest. Get more sleep than you think necessary so that you compensate for the change in your normal sleep cycle. Avoid excess food; don't push yourself physically during the day. Realize that a considerable rest period is needed for you to adjust to the new rhythm. Bear in mind that youths will adjust more readily than those of us who have seen many moons. Flying eastward toward Europe should be followed by a good night's sleep before resuming any significant physical schedule. If you are flying at night, take a morning nap, have a leisurely afternoon, and get to bed early that night. If you're going in the opposite direction by racing the sun across the sky from east to west, go to bed early and sleep for a long time. No matter which direction you are moving, rest is essential for you to recycle your circadian rhythm. The ICAO travel-time formula, as presented in the Air Force *Flight Surgeon's Guide,* is spelled out in Appendix 5. Run through a few examples. Note that the compensation time required is more than you might ordinarily think. But the little extra effort in obtaining adequate rest will pay off in making you a more relaxed, non-fatigued, capable pilot or passenger.

CHAPTER 5

THE EYE, THE EAR, AND HOW THE SENSES LIE

THE MOST IMPORTANT SYSTEMS

Of all the systems of the body, those most important to the flier are the eye, the ear, and the vestibular. The eye is the primary sense on which most dependence must be placed. The ear provides the information from the control tower to the pilot, and the vestibular system produces information necessary for proper orientation in space. The manner in which these systems work, the manner in which they can be exploited if properly understood, and the manner in which they can be damaged if improperly treated, are important for all of us to understand.

THE EYE

"Critical" is the only term adequate to describe the role of the eye in flying. Without good vision, the pilot is lost. Vision is the singular sense on which we must depend for overcoming disorientation.

The eye and its vision sense provide the cues that allow us to do so much in flying. The eye allows us to use the gauges for instrument flying. The eye gives us reference in performing commercial maneuvers such as "pylon eights" and "Immelmans." The eye provides our depth perception, required for good takeoffs and landings. The eye perceives color that is cued in to an "off flag" on our glideslope, to beacons and tower signals, and to map symbols. Most important, the eye provides a "lock-on" for our gauges, which overcomes disorientation due to faulty input of our vestibular and kinesthetic senses. The eye is so critical as a primary sense in flying, it behooves us to know something of ocular, or eye, function —both anatomically and physiologically.

ANATOMY

The eye is, conceptually, a rather simple organ. Think of the eye as a camera with a lens up front and photographic film in the back. The globe or ball of the eye is moved by muscles that can accurately control the eye's position. After patterns of light travel through the lens in the front of the eye, photochemical changes take place in the retina, or film of the eye, in its most posterior or rearward aspect. The photochemical changes create neural impulses that our brain can interpret.

The retina has two separate components: rods and cones. The cones are located in the central portion of the retina—directly behind the lens.

The cones function during daylight and are our primary source of color perception. The rods are located more peripherally along the surface of the retina. They function in diminished illumination (about the level of full moonlight, or .01 foot-candle), and are our primary night visual elements. The rods do not respond accurately to color. Of particular interest is the neural connection of the rods and cones. Each cone is responsible for accurate daylight vision and color perception and has its own nerve element feeding into the brain; however, several rods feed into one neural component. This probably explains why our daylight vision is so much more precise than is our night vision (see Figures 5-1 and 5-2).

Physiology

The physiology of the eye is really related to visibility. The visibility of anything we see depends on: 1. the angular size of the object; 2. the quantity and direction of illumination; 3. the contrast between the object and its background; 4. the length of time it is seen; 5. the degree of retinal adaptation; and 6. the condition of the atmosphere separating the observer and the object. These topics are well explained in an aero-

Figure 5-1
demonstrates the areas of central and peripheral vision. The area of central vision is important since this area is responsible for the most acute vision in adequate light. Even down to a level of moonlight, the central area will function well. In dim light, however, the area of central vision is essentially blind, and we depend upon our area of peripheral vision, which contains the rods of the retina. The area of peripheral vision is critical for vision in dim light. In order to employ this peripheral area, we must remember to scan, since we will otherwise miss what is directly in front of us.

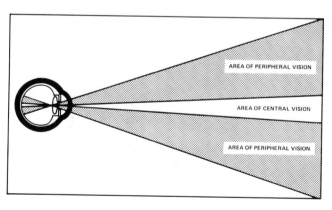

AREA OF PERIPHERAL VISION

AREA OF CENTRAL VISION

AREA OF PERIPHERAL VISION

Figure 5-2
is a breakdown of eye anatomy and
physiology, which focuses on the
major points of interest to the pilot.

EYE ANATOMY AND PHYSIOLOGY

EYE ANATOMY

Retina: back of eye records impulses

		Works During	Color	Locus
1.	Rods	night	no	peripheral
2.	Cones	day	yes	central

EYE PHYSIOLOGY

Vision depends on:
1. angular size
2. illumination
3. contrast
4. time viewed
5. adaptation
6. interface condition

We can compensate for one by varying the other five.

space medicine pamphlet, *Physiology of Flight* (AFP 161-16). I mention this pamphlet because professional pilots will do well to read the entire manual.

The visibility of an object—as you might expect—increases with its angular size, illumination, contrast, viewing time, retinal adaptation and atmospheric clarity. Certainly not an outrageous statement! Of particular interest is that as we diminish or decrease any one of the six factors, the other five factors come into play to compensate for the diminishment of one. For example, an object that is really too small to see under ordinary circumstances can be made visible by increasing the illumination on it or increasing the contrast between the object and its background, or both. On the other hand, if an object cannot be seen because of poor contrast, increase the length of time of viewing and the object becomes visible (e.g., a moving airplane). In the case of a pilot, we know that having an object visible for longer than one second does not significantly increase its

visibility. Therefore, the message from the physiology section is to scan! And scan again!

IllumiNatioN aNd CoNTRasT

An object is more visible as the brightness on it
is increased. In levels of illumination such as on a
heavily overcast day (about 1,000 footcandles), we
have achieved maximum visibility. In fact, at
intense levels of illumination (say 10,000 footcandles), we find it uncomfortable and have to
squint in the glare. At extremes, flash blindness—
an inability to see—develops.

Brightness contrast is an important consideration for all fliers. If we expect our visibility to be
increased by improving our contrast, the best way
we can effect this is to keep our glasses and
windshields clean. Insects, grease, dust, small
particles of dirt—all scatter light, which destroys
the sharpness of the visual image. Fogging or
scratching of our acrylic windshields achieves the
same confusion. The increased reflection of dirty
windshields diminishes light and subsequently
contrast. Furthermore, reflections from a dirty
windshield into the cockpit are distracting as well
as fatiguing. Clean visual surfaces allow for
maximum visibility, illumination, and contrast.
Clean your windshield with a proper plastic
cleaner and a soft nonscratching rag before each
flight. It is your chance on the ground to improve
your performance in the air.

BRiGHTNESS PROTECTiON

The exposure to bright light varies tremen-
dously in a flying environment. We get direct
sunlight, reflections from clouds and water, and
sometimes rapidly changing intensity of light as
we fly into and out of the clouds. A good sunglass

lens is a valuable investment. Several criteria must be met: 1. glasses (or plastic lenses) must not distort; 2. the right and left lenses must be equally matched and must transmit in the visible spectrum within 20 percent of each other; and 3. imperfections that scatter light in the lenses must not be present.

Sunglass Requirements

As a result of extensive studies and in order to meet the varying requirements of sunglasses in the flying environment, criteria have been developed for the "best" sunglasses for a pilot. Sunglasses should eliminate glare by absorbing enough light without decreasing the visual acuity. In technical terms, this has been compromised at about 15 percent. Nonetheless, you can appreciate that wearing sunglasses in low light conditions is bound to decrease object visibility. Sunglasses should not be color distorting. In other words, their color absorption should be essentially neutral. Sunglasses should absorb ultraviolet and infrared radiation, which can be harmful to us. All glass lenses perform this function, but not all plastic lenses do. In short, a glass lens offers better protection, since plastic lenses do not protect against infrared radiation adequately. If you insist on wearing plastic lenses, do not look directly at the sun.

Night Vision

We depend on our rods, or the peripheral elements of the retina, for seeing at night. Color vision at night is difficult and depends on a high intensity of color in order for us to perceive the signal as a color signal. Due to the loss of visual acuity at night, we depend on generalized contours and outlines and not on small distinguishing features. This is a direct consequence of the way the neural elements are gathered in the retina. Remember that several rods feed into one nerve, so that our visual acuity at night is less than during the day. Another important factor is that the rods are located peripherally. Hence, if we look at objects directly at night, we will see them less clearly than if we look at them peripherally or by way of a scan. We are back to the old adage: "Move them eyes."

There are tricks we can play that help us to see better at night. We all recognize that when we go from a bright, sunlit environment into a dark environment, it takes us awhile to begin to see well. This phenomenon is called dark adaptation. Experimentally, we have found that maximum sensitivity of the eye can be achieved after remaining in the dark about 30 minutes. In fact, the sensitivity of our eye increases 10,000-fold during these 30 minutes! Someone has said that under perfect circumstances, a completely dark-adapted eye can detect a match being lit 25 miles away.

There is, however, a great deal of individual variation in adaptation to darkness. We know that people who work in bright sunlight cannot dark-adapt as well as normal individuals can until they have been out of a sunlit environment for several days. To a pilot, this means that bright-sunlight flying during the day is bound to reduce visual acuity at night. The best protection you have for maintaining a good darkness adaptation is to keep your retinal pigments from bleaching out by using sunglass protection when bright sunlight is present.

Aids for Night Vision

While we are on the subject of adaptation to darkness, those of you who spent time in the service already know a trick for assisting visual acuity at night. Wear a red goggle, and darkness adaptation is assisted. The rods, which are our primary night visual receptor, are more sensitive to blue light than to red. Therefore, we wear a red goggle, and this dark-adapts our blue rods (our more sensitive rods). While the adaptation to darkness is not as good as it is in 30 minutes of no light, this compromise allows us to function in an artificially lighted environment and then jump out into the dark, partially adapted.

Oxygen is critical for night vision. At 12,000 feet our night vision is decreased by 50 percent. This is why the military stays on 100 percent oxygen at night. Those of us in general aviation should take a lesson from the people who are in the business of saving their own butts. For sure, use oxygen above 5,000 feet if you are flying at night.

The problem of the effects of hypoxia, or low oxygen, on fliers is compounded by carbon monoxide levels. We know that an ordinary smoker is at a physiological 8,000 feet while still on the ground. Therefore, the smoker is already behind the eight ball before he takes off. Any smoker should maintain himself on oxygen from sea level on up if he wants to have the maximum visual acuity when flying at night.

Finally, comment must be made regarding rabbits' carrot eating. We know from our Nobel Prize winner, George Wald, that rhodopsin, the visual pigment in the retina, is composed largely of vitamin A. Vitamin A is present in carrots, as well as in liver, eggs, cheese, peaches, spinach, and all sorts of greens. These foods should be part of every pilot's well-balanced diet.

Instrument Lighting

How can we use the research that is so abundant to suggest the ideal lighting system for our airplane? We really are caught in a dilemma. We know from the foregoing discussion that we see best in pure white light of adequate intensity to allow our cones to do the seeing. We know that when we look outside the cockpit, the light is dim, and we depend on our rods, whose sensitivity is diminished by bright light. So, we cannot have our cake and eat it too. We cannot have a nice, brightly lit cockpit that shows our instruments to maximum advantage and at the same time be able to function beyond the instrument panel to see what we are going to hit and where we are going to land. So you ask, why not use the old red-light trick? Those of us who have flown at night know that our beautifully colored maps disappear into a black-and-white unintelligible mess under red light. What, then, are the requirements for a good lighting system?

There are several requirements that are important for good instrument lighting: 1. illuminate all important instruments uniformly; 2. do not aim lights directly at the pilot's eyes or in such a way that they might reflect into his eyes; 3. avoid reflections from the windshield or windows; 4. use red light where possible to maximize adaptation to darkness; 5. maintain a light intensity of slightly under 1 footcandle; 6. maintain minimum extraneous light within the cockpit; and 7. keep the lighting sources from obstructing the instruments.

Sounds easy, but we all know that it is not. Since we cannot afford the ultrasophisticated systems that are present in many military aircraft with internally lit individually variable red- and/or white-light sources, we must compromise. Peripherally lit instruments with just enough light to see them without straining are your best bet. Keep a white spotlight on low intensity for reading your maps. Organize your flying so that you do not need to use brighter white light during takeoff and landing sequences. Try keeping one eye closed when using white light.

For those of us misguided enough to get near thunderstorms, remember that the flashes of lightning will blind us if we are totally dark-adapted. Whence cometh the exception. Turn up the lights in your cockpit for all they are worth when you are near thunderstorms. The best protection against flash blindness is a bright cockpit.

Recognition Time

How many of us general aviation pilots ever look at oil-burner routes, or military practice areas, or low-level routes in the *Airman's Information Manual (AIM)*? How many of us even know how to find out if a military low-level route is in action? How many of us even know why this information is important? I owned a small airplane and flew general aviation long before I flew military fighters. I sat on the other side of the fence. Pushing a fighter around at 100 feet AGL (above ground level) at 600 miles per hour ground speed has made me realize how important it is that the average general aviation pilot know how to find out when he is becoming a target whose demise is imminent.

There is a very good reason for the military fighter pilot's practicing low-level routes. The means of getting to the enemy who has been spotted—say, by a forward air-control observer—is to come in on the deck. This maneuver avoids radar lock-on and degrades any SAM missile launch. The routes are usually flown with planes in formations of four. Low-level combat formation usually places the planes several thousand feet apart, zigging and zagging in high-G turns to discourage any ground observers from deciding what the planes' track is going to be and to keep enemy airplanes from having a good idea of just who is where should the formation be jumped.

So the military pilot has his hands full at Mach .95 in high-G turns keeping track of his formation and the hills coming at him at almost supersonic speeds while he flies 100 feet above the ground level. Now, the low-level run extends over a zig-zag course, which finally terminates in an attack on a simulated or real target. The attack is initiated by a pull-up at a defined locus, usually several miles from the target. A high-G climb—frequently 60 degrees above the horizon—is terminated in a pop-up maneuver. This leads to the airplane's—which is now heading toward the heavens—rolling onto its back, lowering its nose while maintaining positive Gs, then rolling wings level and heading in to the target in a 45-degree dive at 450 knots indicated. While all this is happening, bomb racks are being selected, bomb sites are being adjusted, gun switches are being unlocked, the throttle is being adjusted, and all this in between a scan that keeps ASI at 450 knots, attitude precisely at 45 degrees, and altitude of pickle within a fraction of a second. If the airspeed, attitude, and altitude at time of release are not perfect, the bomb misses. Following the pickle, or release of the bomb, the pilot executes a relatively violent maneuver, usually characterized by a hard pull-up of 5 Gs, while the plane is turned either to the left or right to get out of the way of the next in the formation, who is already initiating his bomb run. If you in a small plane are a potential target within this sequence block, you do not achieve A-1 priority status. A fighter pilot has his hands full trying to fly his own plane without worrying about you out there.

Understanding the problems that the military pilot is bound to have and understanding the necessity for his training in these procedures, we as general aviation pilots must realize that the obligation for staying out of these training areas is ours. Military routes are, of course, published in the *AIM*. It is best to ask our flight instructors where they are so that we will know how to avoid these areas. It is best to look at a VFR map and identify landmarks that will help us to avoid these areas. To find out if the areas are active and/or if there is military maneuvering in the area, contact the local flight service station. Before initiating a low-level route, the commander of the fighter squadron will notify flight service station of time and point of entry and the amount of time his formation will be in the block. Critical it is that we as general aviation pilots avoid an area of potential collision. As you can appreciate from the discussion of vision recognition times, the chances of encountering a plane masked by terrain at low level at supersonic speeds can make for an impossible situation. Assuming we see each other (and we may not), the ability to avoid a collision—should that course be so set—may not be present.

Here is the total problem encountered in potential high-speed collisions. While traveling at jet speed, the reaction time, eye movement, foveal perception, accommodation, and recognition are all added up to demonstrate the time taken for

Figure 5-3 demonstrates the early delay in the recognition of an airplane on a collision course with you. After you have fixed your visual axis on an object to be viewed, the physical nature of your fovea or retinal portion of the eye requires a perception time of 0.7 seconds. The total time from extrafoveal appearance to central perception is 0.4 seconds, or a distance traveled of over 1,000 feet. This is merely an early stage in the time delay required to appreciate a potential collision course.

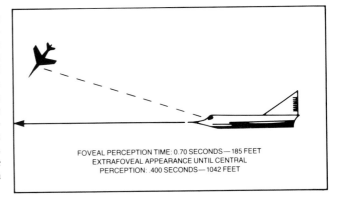

FOVEAL PERCEPTION TIME: 0.70 SECONDS—185 FEET
EXTRAFOVEAL APPEARANCE UNTIL CENTRAL
PERCEPTION: .400 SECONDS—1042 FEET

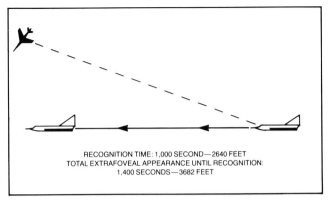

RECOGNITION TIME: 1,000 SECOND—2640 FEET
TOTAL EXTRAFOVEAL APPEARANCE UNTIL RECOGNITION:
1,400 SECONDS—3682 FEET

Figure 5-4
demonstrates an additional stage in the time delay inherent in avoiding a potential collision course. The speed of recognition varies from one individual to the next, but can extend from .65 seconds to 1.5 seconds, averaging about one second for most of us. We now have added another second onto the 0.4 in Figure 5-3. We have traveled almost 4,000 feet toward a collision.

each component and the amount of distance traveled during this time (see Figures 5-3, 5-4 and 5-5). The message should be clear not to put ourselves in a condition where a collision can occur and to react swiftly should the occasion arise. In this case, your plane would have traveled almost one mile (4,050/5,280 feet) before any input to your plane controls could take place.

Reaction Time	.175 seconds =	462 feet
Eye Movement	.050 seconds =	132 feet
Foveal Perception	.070 seconds =	185 feet
Accommodation	.500 seconds =	1,320 feet
Recognition	.800 seconds =	1,952 feet
Total 1.6	seconds =	4,050 feet

Figure 5-5
demonstrates the bottom line of a potential collision course. If we were to emerge at jet speeds from clouds 3,000 feet apart, already on a collision course, we would crash before we could do anything about it. If, in fact, the distance were only 500 feet, we would never have time to see each other before we crashed. In view of the mix of commercial and military jet traffic, accompanied by slower general aviation traffic, we can appreciate the inherent danger when flying close to clouds, when entering areas of oil-burner routes or restricted military zones, and/or when mixing traffic in airport control zones. The one way to avoid a disaster is to keep your head out of the cockpit as much as possible, obey the "rules of the road" with regard to maintaining altitude and position, and react swiftly when you anticipate a problem.

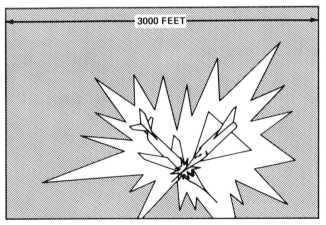

3000 FEET

Tips for Better Vision

Let us put together some of what we have said with further expansion to allow us to see better. We have made a big plea to "scan." But a little knowledge is a dangerous thing. We can see fine material by looking directly at it. For example, offset your eye about 10 degrees from the edge of this book and try to read. Everything disappears. We know that we have to be looking directly at something to read it. That means if we are too busy scanning rapidly, we may see nothing. This is close to the truth. By scanning, we mean a series of short, jerky, movements—not a large sweep. What is true of this printed material is also true of airplanes outside your cockpit. We do not see them by sweeping the sky in a rapid, even manner. We see them by sweeping the sky in short bursts of scan. Scan indeed! But scan with short interval movements.

Now how about judging distance in depth? There are many clues we can use to improve our perception of distance and depth. Ordinarily, we depend unconsciously on interplay between our two eyes. This binocular vision provides for an unconscious measure of distance and depth dependent upon our past experience. There are lots of other clues that we can use that are monocular or single-eye clues. For example, geometric perspective changes as we near an object. We know that if one object overlaps another, the second or overlapped object is farther away. We know that if a shadow is seen nearer our cockpit than is the object, then the object is nearer than the light. Our perspective teaches us that objects that are seen less clearly tend to be farther away. Terrestrial association is helpful. For example, an airplane turning final with its wheels down can be thought of as being at the same distance as the particular airport at which it is landing. And, finally, motion parallax teaches us that when we move our head, an object moving in the distance is farther away than the one nearer us, which appears fixed. What I am suggesting is that we can train ourselves to use clues around us that are helpful in determining depth and distance. Do not take them for granted!

A clean canopy is a prerequisite for safe flight. A dirty or crazed canopy diminishes vision and scatters light—sometimes blinding the pilot. A preparation such as Meguiar's Mirror Glaze should be employed to clean plastic windshields. *Make certain to use a soft, nonscratching cloth.*

Here is a series of tips for improving day and night vision:

Tips for Day Seeing

1. Scan in bursts.
2. Clean your windshield.
3. Wear good sunglasses on bright days.
4. Develop monocular clues for depth.

Tips for Night Seeing

1. Use side vision.
2. Dark adapt.
3. Use oxygen.
4. Eat like a rabbit.
5. Minimal instrument lighting.
6. Avoid bright light during landing and takeoff.
7. Use bright light in thunderstorms.

Ocular Illusions

We have discussed illusions in the spatial orientation section (Chapter 3). It would not do to forget the ocular illusions, lest we believe that everything we see with our eyes allows us to fly properly. Autokinesis is the most frequent optic illusion. If we stare at a light that is fixed in position, in a dark environment, the light will tend to move. We can get around this apparent movement-illusion by scanning. Do not pick out a star, a light on a building, or a light on an airplane and stare at it. Move those eyes!

Second, a size–distance illusion appears from staring at a light that is approaching and receding from you. Depth perception becomes difficult! The solution, once again, is to move those eyes!

Sensory illusions are further discussed in Appendix 7.

The Ear

The ear can be divided into three portions: the outer ear, the middle ear, and the inner ear (see Figure 5-6).

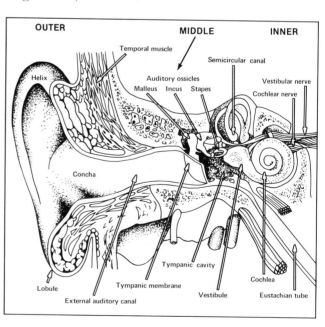

Figure 5-6
illustrates the three portions of the ear: the outer ear, extending from the auricle (helix, concha, and lobule) to the eardrum, or tympanic membrane; the middle ear, extending from the tympanic membrane to the oval window of the cochlea, or inner ear; and the inner ear, containing the sensory components responsible for hearing and vestibular perception. Note that the eustachian tube empties from the middle ear into the nasopharynx, or back of the nose.

OUTER EAR

The outer ear is that part of the ear that we see when we look at an individual. The outer ear extends from the auricle, or visible portion of the ear, through the ear canal to the eardrum or tympanic membrane. The problems encountered in flying that can affect the outer ear are confined to diseases and mechanical obstruction. Diseases of the outer ear vary from frostbite to infection. Should the ear become swollen or painful, or should you feel your hearing has diminished, your AME should be consulted. The most common mechanical obstruction in the outer ear is cerumen, or wax. You should not try to clean your own outer ear with cotton swabs or other devices. Outer ears are self-cleaning; should they obstruct, the cleansing is a job for the physician and not for you. I cannot even speculate on the number of injuries I have seen to both the ear canal and the eardrum from pilots whose attempt to cleanse the ear led to a complication that was totally avoidable.

Middle Ear

The middle ear is that portion of the ear structure between the eardrum and the sensorineural components of the inner ear (see Figure 2-22 on page 66). The middle ear is an air-filled cavity, which contains the three ossicles, or ear bones, and is connected to the back of the nose, or nasopharynx, by the eustachian tube. The middle ear is the portion of the ear most commonly affected during flying, especially during descents. When there is obstruction to the eustachian tube drainage, or aeration of the middle ear, a negative pressure develops in the middle ear. If this pressure is not relieved by swallowing or by a Valsalva maneuver, fluid takes the space of the air in the middle ear (see Figure 2-24 on page 66). When there is obstruction and thence fluid, be it in the lung, kidney, or other organ of the body, infection follows. Pain develops; the eardrum ruptures. The secret to maintaining a healthy middle ear is to maintain good aeration. This means that you should not fly when there is any obstruction to eustachian-tube drainage or aeration, such as when you have a cold. This means that you should descend slowly enough so that you can properly aerate the middle ear (see Figure 2-23 on page 66). Keep swallowing. If necessary, hold your nose, blow with mouth closed and swallow again; this is a Valsalva maneuver. Furthermore, a negative pressure in the middle ear space has an adverse effect on inner ear function; abnormal pressures adversely affect hearing and equilibrium. Thus, an improperly aerated or diseased middle ear is a set-up for inner ear dysfunction, which, should it affect the vestibular system, can be disastrous to a pilot. As noted in Chapter 3, the consequence of a middle ear block can be a paracentesis or drainage of the middle ear by placing a pinhole in the eardrum itself. For the most part, however, decongestant medication will usually clear up both an ear block (fluid or negative air pressure) and/or infection. The point is to see your AME early whenever you feel that any problem exists in your ear. The ear is too critical an organ, on the ground or in the air, for you to take chances or procrastinate regarding care. Get some advice early in the game before a permanent problem develops.

Inner Ear

The inner ear is the fluid-filled sensorineural portion of the ear, which is responsible for converting mechanical impulses from the outer and

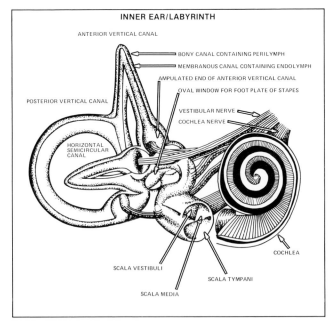

INNER EAR/LABYRINTH

ANTERIOR VERTICAL CANAL

BONY CANAL CONTAINING PERILYMPH
MEMBRANOUS CANAL CONTAINING ENDOLYMPH
AMPULATED END OF ANTERIOR VERTICAL CANAL
OVAL WINDOW FOR FOOT PLATE OF STAPES

POSTERIOR VERTICAL CANAL

VESTIBULAR NERVE
COCHLEA NERVE

HORIZONTAL
SEMICIRCULAR
CANAL

COCHLEA

SCALA VESTIBULI

SCALA TYMPANI

SCALA MEDIA

middle ear into electro-chemical and, thus, sensory pulses that can be interpreted by the brain. (See Figure 5-7.)

Ear Physiology

The physiology of the entire ear mechanism is easily understood: sound waves enter the ear canal, where speech frequencies (about 1,000 Hz or cycles per second) are funneled through the ear canal much as they would be in a resonating organ pipe. The sound impulses hit the tympanic membrane or eardrum, then vibrate the three ear bones, which have a lever, or amplification, factor of 1.3. Sound carried by transmission of these ear bones then vibrates the inner ear fluid. The ratio of the size of the eardrum to the oval window of the inner ear into which the third ear bone or stapes is centered is 17 to 1. When this ratio is multiplied by the 1.3 lever effect of the

Figure 5-7 illustrates the inner ear. The inner ear can be divided into two portions: the *cochlea*, responsible for hearing, and the labyrinth (*semicircular canals* and *maculae*), responsible for balance. The cochlea is divided into three parts: the scala vestibuli, scala media, and scala tympani. These three portions are stimulated by sound transmissions entering through the oval window from the foot plate of the stapes. Impulses generated by hair cells within the cochlea are fed out the cochlear nerve into the brain. The labyrinthine balance system consists of three semicircular canals—the horizontal, posterior, and anterior canals. These three canals are oriented in three different planes so as to perceive angular motion in their respective planes. The macula acustica, or sense organ of the utricle, and saccule are responsible for appreciating linear acceleration such as G forces. The semicircular canals, saccule, and utricle are encased within a bony canal containing perilymph, in which is placed a membranous canal containing endolymph. The difference in ion potentials between the endolymph and perilymph creates the biochemical electrical impulses passed on through the nerves. The vestibular nerve is responsible for conducting pulses to the brain to allow us to maintain our state of balance.

ossicles, the total amplification of the filtered outer and middle ear systems is approximately 20 to 1. This amplified sound then extends into the fluid of the inner ear, where special sensory hair cells of the inner ear are stimulated at appropriate levels (depending upon the frequency of the sound) and converted into neural impulses. Electrical nerve pulses are then sent topside, where the brain puts together the pattern of sound and frequencies that leads to our interpretation.

Based on this description, it is apparent that both the outer and middle ear are mechanical structures for which surgical remedy is almost always available. The inner ear, on the other hand, is a very fragile neurosensory structure for which no surgical reconstruction is possible. The consequences of this logic is that damage to the inner ear is usually permanent and thus IRREVERSIBLE. This is an important consideration, since the primary damage to the inner ear in fliers is caused by either rapid pressure changes or, in most cases, by loud noise.

INNER EAR DAMAGE

Rapid pressure changes can actually result in a leak of fluid from the inner ear out into the middle ear. If this leakage does not stop and/or is not sealed off surgically at its exit into the middle ear, permanent—and usually total—hearing loss will result. The damage to the inner ear from loud sound is well documented in the population at large and in fliers in particular. How many of us have seen a middle-aged pilot who cups his hand over his ear and says, "Say again"? We immediately think to ourselves "Aha! An old B-17 pilot." But the damage from noise to our inner ears is not peculiar to the man who rumbled around World War II in a loud airplane. It is a vocational and an avocational disorder of virtually all pilots, because almost all airplanes have a loudness exceeding government-accepted standards for noise levels even in industry.

BAROMETRIC CHANGES

We have all noticed the effect of barometric pressure changes on our ears. As we ascend, the air pressure around us decreases. The consequence is that the pressure inside the middle ear increases. One of two things must then happen: either the pressure builds up to the point where it ruptures the eardrum, or the eustachian tube opens and allows release of this pressure. We sense the eustachian tube's opening to relieve the pressure at approximately 15 mm of mercury. This forces a small bubble of air down the eustachian tube and into the back of our nose. We sense this as a release of fullness in the ear, usually accompanied by a click. When we descend, however, the pressure changes in the ear must reverse.

We have all noticed that the effect of descending is greatest nearest the earth. It is the last few thousand feet that produce the greatest pressure differential. For example, if we descend from a high altitude to, say, 15,000 feet, we will have almost no discomfort regardless of the rate of descent. This is one of the reasons the military can allow their pilots who have ejected to free-fall without any sequelae to the ear to 15,000 feet before their parachute opens. However, if we descend another 10,000 feet, discomfort is likely.

The Germans during World War II understood the problem of equalizing pressure at low altitudes. They punctured holes in their dive-bomber pilots' eardrums and frequently put in small metal tubes to allow rapid pressure changes without the pilots' having to swallow. This, of course, produced dive bombing without any chance of pilot incapacitation due to pain and/or vertigo from inability to equalize the pressure. A simple extention of the principle of swallowing and/or yawning to equalize the pressure in the ears is the rationale for waking a sleeping passenger prior to descent in a commercial airliner. We seldom yawn or swallow while we are sleeping. Therefore, we are more susceptible to an ear block if we go through the last thousand feet while asleep. Thus the flight attendant walks around tickling our chins to mobilize us into a position where an ear block will not develop.

Because of the influx of turbocharged airplanes into the general aviation inventory and the tendency for so much of our commercial flight to take place at higher altitudes, it is worth discussing the problems associated with breathing oxygen and the middle ear. When we saturate our middle ear space by breathing oxygen and then land, the oxygen is subsequently used up by the mucous membrane, or tissue, of the middle ear. This leads to negative pressure. If we swallow and blow, this pressure will normally be cleared. However, if it is at night and we go to bed, the oxygen may be reabsorbed and when we wake up we are left with an ear block, perhaps painful. Thus, a tip—if we have been on 100 percent oxygen and we land and are not going to be awake for several hours, Valsalva several times and consider spraying your nose with decongestant medication such as Otrivin or Afrin, which will shrink the membranes and allow the eustachian tube to equilibrate more readily. Warning—do not get into the habit of using any nasal vasoconstrictor, such as Neo-Synephrine, chronically. The results can be catastrophic on both the nasal mucous membranes and on the sinuses that empty onto them. To maintain good aeration, here are rules to follow:

- Do not fly with a cold or hay fever.
- Descend slowly enough to clear middle ear.
- Swallow and/or chew gum on descent.
- Use Valsalva maneuver to open eustachian tubes.
- If an ear block develops, reascend and spray nose with decongestant.

COMMUNICATION

The inner ear's primary function is communication. It is to this end that the major portion of our discussion must be directed. Effective communication is the sine qua non of safe, controlled air travel. I trained on a 1,600-foot-long, nine-foot-wide strip adjacent to two large commercial airports. I had 200 hours under my belt before I had to give any serious thought to using a radio. But *today* is terminal control zones and requirements for transponders, and all the rest of the government regulations. It is naive for any of us to think that the good old days, with seat-of-the-pants, out-of-your-backyard flying, are going to be the rule any longer. Quite to the contrary, they have to be the exception. We have all heard the story of the commercial airline pilot who departed Logan Airport only to be asked by the departure controller, "Say altitude." The pilot: "Altitude." The controller: "I say again, say altitude." The reply: "Altitude." Controller: "Say, 'Canceling IFR.'" Effective communication is a must if we are going to keep our environment safe and mutually understand what we are expected to do.

How, then, can our understanding of the inner ear assist us in understanding problems associated with communication? First, we must protect our ears. The single best way to protect our ears is to use headphones (see Figure 4-10 on p. 114). These serve to increase effective communication by including the communication set within them, and also serve to protect our ears from harmful noise with a fluid-filled earmuff seal. We can accomplish a similar, albeit smaller, effect by not running our radios louder than necessary. If we find the cost of earphones too great and/or the systems within the plane not readily adaptable to earphones, we can gain much of the same protection by using earplugs (see Figure 4-7 on p. 113).

The problem of communication in a noisy aircraft cockpit is compounded by tricks the ear can play upon us. The auditory system has been designed to discriminate only the better of two sounds. More simply put, we will hear only the louder of two sounds. This provides us with stereophonic sound localization. It also eliminates a lot of extraneous sounds on which we might not want to concentrate. The problem with this system is that the quieter sounds will be totally rejected, i.e., not heard at all by our brain. Let's take an example.

We are in a landing pattern. We have been told to keep up our airspeed because American Airlines is sitting behind us. We turn base while throwing out flaps and the gear, which we have suddenly remembered with the onset of noise and vibration. At that very instant, the controller says, "62AH on collision course with military A-10, turn right—now!" We all know that "now" means NOW, but our gear and our flaps and our burble are louder than the "NOW." And the inevitable results. This could, of course, have been avoided with proper noise protection such as earphones and earmuffs. The fact is that we only hear the better of two sounds. The trick in flying is to make sure we hear the right sounds and not the noise.

The sequelae of not protecting our ears is sensorineural hearing loss. Take a gander at Figure 4-6 (p. 112). The high tones go first; then all the tones go. The effect of aging or presbycusis are compounded by the effects of noise damage on the ear. The result is a 40-year-old pilot who cannot communicate effectively. Every pilot should wear ear protection while he or she is flying.

HOW THE SENSES LIE

Our ability to determine where we are is dependent upon the integration of inputs by our brain from the vestibular sense, the propriocep-tive sense, and the visual sense. These three senses are integrated in order to allow us to orient ourselves in space and to keep from being motion sick. The vestibular sense is the input from the inner ear, which tells us whether we are up, down, and/or spinning. The proprioceptive, or kinesthetic sense, is the old seat-of-the-pants sense, which comes from sensory receptors in our skin and joints. The visual sense has been discussed in the first part of this chapter and is the primary sense on which we must depend in flying aircraft. In order for us to understand better how deceptive the vestibular-proprioceptive input can be, we must first understand the anatomy and physiology of this input. Then we can better extrapolate the vestibular sense role in spatial disorientation and motion sickness.

ANATOMY

The inner ear apparatus, which we have discussed in the second part of this chapter, is divided into two portions: the *cochlea*, which is responsible for auditory or hearing function, and the *labyrinth*, which is responsible for vestibular, or position-sense, function. The labyrinth may be thought of as composed of two portions: 1. the saccule and utricle, which are responsible for sensing up and down or G forces; and 2. the three semicircular canals responsible for monitoring angular acceleration or turning. The three semicircular canals lie in three different planes so that the fluid within them will be stimulated by angular acceleration in one of three planes.

The utricle and saccule, which are responsible for detecting linear acceleration, are small membranous sacs with microscopic hairs protruding into them. These microscopic hairs hold up a gelatin structure, which contains small calcium particles. As the calcium particles imbedded in the gel shift with linear acceleration, the small hair endings are deformed, stimulated, and send a

Figure 5-8
is a schematic of a microscopic cross section of the sensory receptor (macula) of the utricle or saccule. The otoliths or calcium particles are embedded in a gelatinous layer that rests against the filaments of hair cells. It is these hair cells that, when deformed, provide the biochemical potential that is transmitted by way of the medulated nerve fibers as action potentials by the vestibular nerve into the brain. This macula is responsible for sensing linear acceleration or G forces.

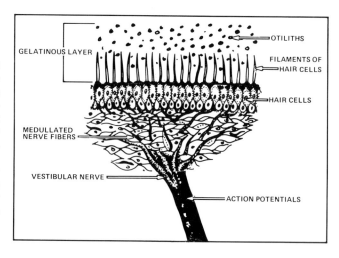

neural impulse that we interpret as a linear
acceleration or G force (see Figure 5-8).

The anatomy and function of the semicircular
canals is conceptually very similar to that of the
utricle and saccule. At the base of each semicircular canal is an expanded saccular structure
called the ampulla. Into the ampulla project
small hairs, which are directly stimulated by the
flow of fluid in the semicircular canal itself. As in
the utricle, deformation of these microscopic
hairs then generates a neural pulse, which is
projected to the brain, where we interpret the
impulses as motion (see Figure 5-9).

The inner ear does not exist in a vacuum but
interrelates with other sensory systems such as the
cerebellum of the brain, into which most of the
proprioceptive senses feed. There are many neural systems that interact to compensate for vestibular information. For years neurophysiologists
have attempted to establish a model that could
adequately explain this interrelationship. This
author, in 1968, presented a paper, based upon
neurological experiments in many animals, to
the Aerospace Medical Association. For those of
you interested in understanding the vestibular
system in more depth, we have included this
schematic model in Figure 5-10.

Figure 5-9
is a schematic microscopic cross section of the sensory organ (ampulla)
of the semicircular canal. The fluid
(endolymph) is stimulated by angular acceleration to move against the
cupula. Movement of the cupula
stimulates hair cells, which by way
of a biochemical reaction leads to
action potentials that are carried
down the medulated nerve fibers,
through the vestibular nerve and
into the brain. Note the structural
similarity of the cupula hair cell
complex in the semicircular canal to
that of the macula in the otolith
organs schematized in Figure 5-8.

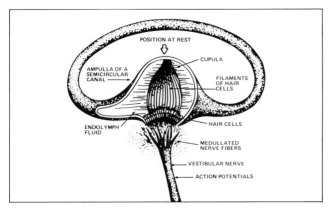

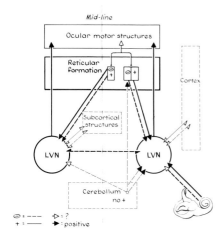

Figure 5-10
is a schematic model of the interrelation of the semicircular canals with other neural systems. The semicircular canals feed into the lateral vestibular nucleus (LVN). Thence, connections project to the reticular formation, which is responsible for alertness and thence to the ocularmotor structures providing compensatory eye movements (nystagmus). The lateral vestibular nuclei are, of course, interrelated so that one canal knows what the other is doing. Projections from the lateral vestibular nuclei also extend to the cortex of the brain, where we sense the subsequent vertigo, and to the cerebellum, where the vestibular input is integrated with impulses coming from the seat-of-the-pants, or proprioceptive, senses. One can imagine the number of parameters to be considered in analyzing such a black box system.

Physiology

The physiology of the vestibular end organ (utricle, saccule, and semicircular canals) is easy to understand if two basic principles of physics are applied: 1. Velocity is a constant rate of speed; and 2. There is a difference between linear and angular motion (see Figure 5-11). We can relate linear speed to a common, everyday situation,

Figure 5-11
illustrates the difference between angular and linear acceleration and the respective vestibular sensory organs that are thereby stimulated. Angular acceleration impacts on the semicircular canals of the vestibular organ, which can be affected by angular acceleration in any of three planes. It is rotatory motion that stimulates the semicircular canals. Linear acceleration, or G forces, on the other hand, affect the utricle and saccule. The combination of semicircular canals and otolith (saccule and utricle) organs provide us with sensory information as to our position.

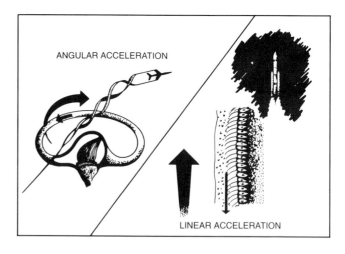

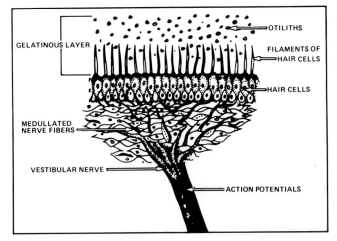

Figure 5-12
schematically demonstrates the situation in the otolith organs (saccule and utricle) when a person is holding his head upright. The normal G force placed upon us on the earth's surface results in a constant, slow discharge into our brain, carried through the otolith nerve. This constant discharge is a function of stimulation by the weight of the otoliths on the filaments of the hair cells and the resultant action potentials carried through the vestibular nerves. When we change our head position, a situation develops as illustrated in Figure 5-13.

such as miles per hour in our car. Angular velocity, unlike linear velocity, represents a constant rotary motion. Since we know that a velocity is a constant rate of speed, if we change the speed, we must apply acceleration or deceleration. We must either increase or decrease the velocity. It is the *change* in velocity—the acceleration or deceleration—that our inner ears detect. Once we are traveling at a constant rate of speed—be it Mach I or 20 mph—our inner ears do not respond.

The distinction between linear and angular acceleration allows us to understand why the utricle and saccule respond differently from the three semicircular canals. Look first at the utricle and saccule (see Figures 5-12 and 5-13). The orientation of the membranes is organized in such a manner that almost any *linear* acceleration will deform the hairs over which the calcium particles are suspended in gel. Experiments have shown that the mechanism of this organ is so finely tuned that a change of only 1.5 degrees in the direction of linear acceleration or of 0.01 G can be detected. A truly remarkable sensory system!

Figure 5-13
schematically demonstrates what happens when we tilt our head or have a G force applied to us, as in straight forward acceleration. The calcium particles, or otoliths, are pulled backward by their inertia, thus pulling the gelatinous layer, which is attached to the filaments of the hair cells. The deformation of the filaments results in an increase in the discharge from the hair cells, which is thence carried as action potentials in the vestibular nerve and interpreted by our brain, appropriately, as acceleration or a change in head position.

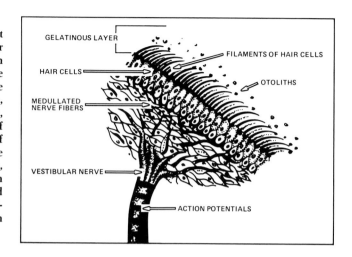

The three semicircular canals do not respond to the linear acceleration for which the saccule and utricle are designed. They respond only to changes in *angular* velocity. As the angular velocity or rotation of the head in plane changes, the fluid in the semicircular canals flows against the hair cells in the ampulla of that canal. As the body achieves a constant rotation, the fluid rotates at the same speed as the body. Then the hair cells return to normal and there is no sensory input. Once the body stops, the fluid continues to spin in the canal, thus stimulating the hair cells

Figure 5-14
illustrates the end organ of the semicircular canal with no stimulus applied. The semicircular canal functions to detect angular acceleration and deceleration. The endolymph fluid at rest offers no stimulus to the cupula; cupula position at rest is straight up. Once angular acceleration is applied to the field, deformation of the cupula will take place as a function of velocity of stimulation and time in seconds or duration of stimulation. It is short-duration stimuli to which the semicircular canals respond most accurately. The next three figures show how the semicircular canals function schematically.

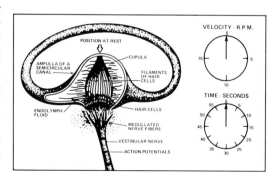

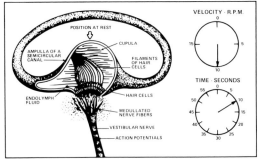

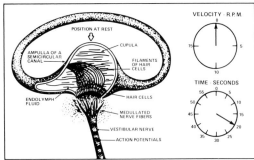

Figure 5-15
demonstrates the effect upon the cupula of 10 revolutions per minute at the 10-second mark. Note the cupula has shifted from its position at rest in Figure 5-14 to a leftward position because of motion of the endolymph fluid in a clockwise direction. This has resulted in stimulation of the hair cells and a consequent action potential carried by the vestibular nerve to our brains. We now know that we are turning.

Figure 5-16
shows the extension of the acceleration or deceleration stimulus to the semicircular canal. We have now stopped turning, and our velocity is zero. Nonetheless, the fluid in the ear canal is now turning at its maximum, and at the 20-second interval the cupula is even more deformed than it was at the 10-second mark noted in Figure 5-15. Thus the stimulus to our brain is even greater. So even though our body has stopped moving, the semicircular canals still serve to function and relate what is happening to our body.

again. This schema is shown in Figures 5-14 through 5-18.

As you might expect, minimal detection of angular acceleration or deceleration is dependent upon the *amount* of angular acceleration to the inner ear and the *time* over which the acceleration is applied. A physiological rule has been established that says the acceleration and the time over which the acceleration is applied when multiplied together must be greater than 2.5 degrees per second to be detectible. For example, if we yawed an airplane (a horizontal angular acceleration) for one second, we would just be able to detect this yaw if the angular acceleration were greater than 2.5 degrees per second. We can play with these numbers ad infinitum. The bottom line is that the semicircular canals are incredibly sensitive.

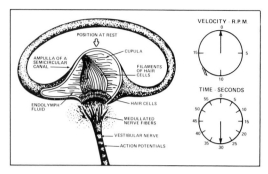

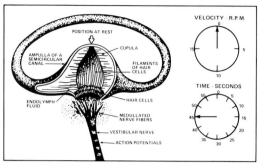

Figure 5-17
demonstrates what is happening to the cupula at the 30-second mark now that our body has stopped moving and our velocity is zero. The cupula is beginning to return to its resting position and the endolymph fluid, because of the sudden stoppage of rotation of our body, has begun circulating in the reverse or counterclockwise direction. Thus, the semicircular canal continues to provide us with information 10 seconds after all motion of the body has stopped. This information can be erroneous. We may feel that we are still rotating because of the semicircular input into the brain.

Figure 5-18
demonstrates the condition of the cupula 45 seconds after initiating the stimulus of rotation. The cupula has now returned to its midline or resting position, and the endolymph fluid is in essentially a static state and not stimulating the cupula. We are back to a condition of a resting discharge from our semicircular canal end organ. This steady-state situation is achieved even if the body has continued to rotate, because the speed of the fluid circulating in the semicircular canal eventually comes to equal the speed of the body rotating. Thus, if we were 40 seconds into a constant rotation without any angular acceleration or deceleration being imposed anew, we would perceive ourselves as not rotating at all, since semicircular canals would be providing no new input to our brain. This static situation is discussed further in the section on spatial disorientation.

THE Coriolis Effect

Understanding the mechanism of semicircular canal function allows us to appreciate the Coriolis effect. We have all experienced the Coriolis effect in disorientation trainers and/or while under the hood with flight instructors. We put our head in our lap with eyes closed; the instructor turns the airplane in a circle: we lift our head fast and open our eyes; the world falls apart. We are convinced that we are upside-down, inside-out, and going every which way. The mechanism for the Coriolis effect is easy to understand.

Whenever one set of semicircular canals has equilibrated to a constant angular velocity, and a rapid head motion is made in a plane different from that equilibration, an immediate angular acceleration is imposed upon another set of semicircular canals. While this angular acceleration is being imposed on the new set of canals, an immediate deceleration takes place on the canals that had previously been equilibrated. Something has to give. Since the semicircular canals are encased on bone and do not provide for immediate deformation compensation, our brain is fed incorrect information, which we find confusing, creating a topsy-turvy feeling, and which sometimes can produce nausea and vomiting.

Nystagmus

By now you are probably asking how we know so much about the vestibular system. As the fluid within the semicircular canals rotates, it stimulates the eyes to compensate by rotating with the fluid. Of course, the eyes cannot turn in a

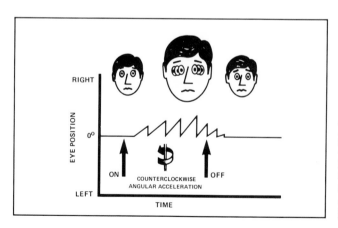

Figure 5-19 schematically represents vestibular nystagmus. Nystagmus is characterized by rapid oscillating movements of the eyes, which follow the fluid movement in the semicircular canals. As the semicircular canal fluid rotates counterclockwise, so will the eyes. As the eyes hit the end of their point of gaze, they will snap back to the midline and begin the rotation anew. This oscillation of slow, fast, slow, fast is called nystagmus. The purpose of nystagmus, of course, is to focus an image on the retina in spite of angular motion imposed on the body. Nystagmus can be thought of as an exaggeration of the compensatory vestibular-ocular reflex. Nystagmus generates an electrical potential that can be recorded, much as a heart tracing in an electrocardiogram; this tracing is called an electronystagmogram and is shown in **Figure 5-21.**

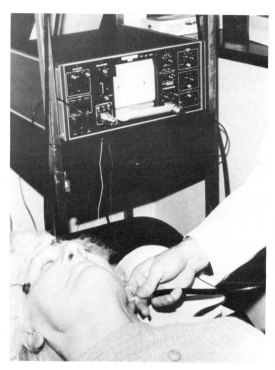

Figure 5-20
is a photograph of the clinical arrangement used in taking an electronystagmogram. Hot or cold water (20cc) is automatically introduced into a patient's ear canal while the patient is 30 degrees to the horizontal. This places the semicircular canals in a vertical plane. The convection of either hot or cold causes the endolymph fluid in the semicircular canal to rotate either up or down and thus stimulate the cupula. The resultant nystagmus from the vestibular organ stimulus is recorded on paper for analysis.

complete circle. When they reach the end of the visual scan, they pop back to a central position and again begin their tracking rotation. This results in periodic eye movements, nystagmus (see Figure 5-19). Nystagmus has a slow, rotating component followed by a fast, jerky, compensatory movement. The slow, rotating movement is generated from the inner ear, while the fast, jerky, compensatory movement is generated by other portions of the brain. Since the eye has a positive potential (much like the heart), we can record electrically the nystagmus and thus study the effects of positioning the pilot under experimental conditions. The ultimate recording (see Figures 5-20 and 5-21) is an electronystagmogram. Nystagmus is the vestibular-ocular reflex that compensates for information from the inner ear.

ELECTRONYSTAGMOGRAM

NAME: _____ DATE: _____

AGE: _____ SEX: _____ EXAMINER: _____ PRE-OP: _____ POST-OP: _____

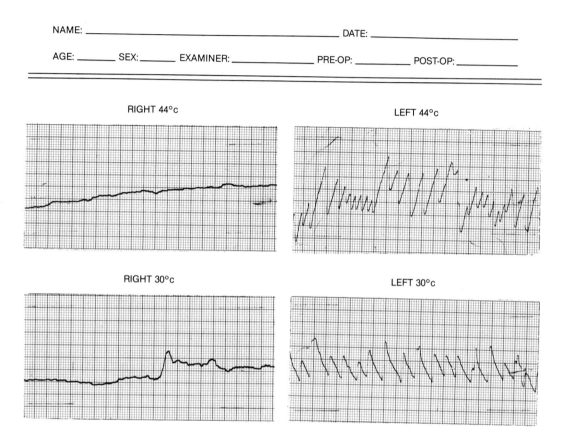

RIGHT 44°c   LEFT 44°c

RIGHT 30°c   LEFT 30°c

Figure 5-21
is an electronystagmogram tracing. Microvolt potentials, picked up by electrodes taped adjacent to the eye, pick up and amplify nystagmus, or movements of the eyes. Eye movements are caused by stimulation of the vestibular system. The output from the electrodes is translated into a heat pen, which makes the tracing called the electronystagmogram. The pilot in this electronystagmogram reported that he was dizzy when making rapid position changes. The weakness of the output from stimulation on the right side has demonstrated a tumor in his vestibular, or balance, nerve. (Ordinarily, a response elicited by flushing hot or cold into either ear would be identical.) The electronystagmogram is similar to an electrocardiogram and is very valuable for evaluating the balance system.

The electronystagmogram provides that vestibular system information.

Kinesthetic Sense

One last comment regarding the proprioceptive or kinesthetic sense. All higher forms of animal life must understand the position of different parts of their body in order to function effectively (see Figure 5-22). We humans integrate a series of receptors beneath our skin with receptors in our muscles, and with receptors in our joints. All three inputs come to the spinal cord, where they feed to the cerebellum of the brain and are there integrated with our vestibular and ocular senses. It is this kinesthetic or proprioceptive sense that allows for seat-of-the-pants flying.

Spatial Disorientation

We have all experienced spatial disorientation. We know that we cannot completely depend upon our vestibular and proprioceptive input to

Figure 5-22
schematically demonstrates the input of the proprioceptive, or kinesthetic, sense. This "seat-of-the-pants" sense is a function of input from (A) the Pacinian corpuscles within the muscles themselves; (B) the neuromuscular spindles contained in the muscles; (C) the Golgi tendon organs located where muscles attach to bone; and, finally, (D) the joint receptors themselves located within the moveable joints of the body. These four inputs provide us with a proprioceptive sense, which tells us where our limbs are and what pressures are being imposed upon them.

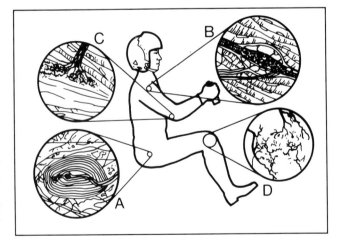

tell us where we are and how we are getting there. We must have input that bypasses the illusions created by the vestibular—proprioceptive senses. This input is visual and comes from reference either to the horizon or to our instruments. Failure to believe our eyes results in spatial disorientation.

Spatial disorientation evolves from both vestibular and nonvestibular causes. Let us look first at vestibular illusions.

The *leans* is the most common form of vestibular spatial disorientation. The basic reason for this illusion is that the semicircular canals allow certain motions to remain unperceived while causing the perception of angular motions that do not even exist. For example, if we are accelerating an airplane four degrees per second for a fraction of a second—say a quarter of a second—a constant angular velocity roll of 1.25 degrees per second results. We know from our physiology discussion that we must have at least 2.5 degrees per second before we recognize the roll. Now let us keep the airplane rolling at the same rate, realizing now that we do not even know that it is rolling. In half a minute we have achieved almost a 40-degree bank. Now let us assume that we are "in the soup." All of a sudden our scan brings us back to our attitude indicator. We make a rapid correction to take out the bank, but this rapid correction is readily perceived by the semicircular canals. In fact, we are now correcting at a rate of more than the magic number of 2.5 degrees per second. As we roll back to the true horizontal, we now perceive the motion. As our attitude indicator comes straight and level, we are left with one of two options. If we are not well instrument trained, we will roll back in the direction of the original unperceived roll to compensate for information coming from our semicircular canals. If we are well instrument trained, we will believe our eyes and keep the airplane straight and level. But we will actually lean our body in the direction of the original roll to compensate for the input from our semicircular canals. The moral to this long song and dance is to believe your gauges. The vestibular system will input false information because of its physical limits. If you think you are moving in a particular direction and your gauges indicate differently—believe your gauges (see Figures 5-23 and 5-24).

Another vestibular illusion easy to understand is the *graveyard spin,* or a *spiral.* We have made a big point of saying that the inner ear responds only to changes in acceleration. Once a constant velocity has been achieved, the ears cannot respond. So if, while disoriented, you put your airplane into a constant spin, the fluid movement in your inner ear will in 20 to 30 seconds catch up with the spinning airplane and stop stimulating

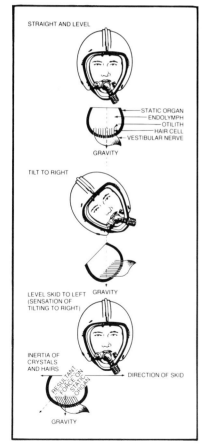

STRAIGHT AND LEVEL

STATIC ORGAN
ENDOLYMPH
OTILITH
HAIR CELL
VESTIBULAR NERVE

GRAVITY

TILT TO RIGHT

LEVEL SKID TO LEFT GRAVITY
(SENSATION OF
TILTING TO RIGHT)

INERTIA OF
CRYSTALS
AND HAIRS

DIRECTION OF SKID

RESULTANT FORCE ON STATIC ORGAN

GRAVITY

Figure 5-23
demonstrates the effect of head position on the stimulus we receive from the macula, contained in the saccule or utricle. The static organ of the saccule or utricle has endolymph fluid in which is suspended a series of otoliths, or calcium particles. These particles rest on a gelatin over hair cells, which, when deformed, will stimulate the vestibular nerve. When we are in a straight-and-level configuration (such as in the top drawing), only a resting discharge, which will give us an awareness of a central head position, will be found. On the other hand, if we tilt our head to the right, gravity will pull the otoliths down and send an impulse to our brain that we will sense as a shift of our head position. The problem with the vestibular system is that illusions can be created in a flying atmosphere. If the plane is level, but skidding to the left, the resultant force on our end organ will seem to us a tilt to the right. This is one of the stimuli that can be responsible for the sensation of the leans. The macular end organ system was designed for terrestrial dwellers. In an airplane we must beware of the information it provides.

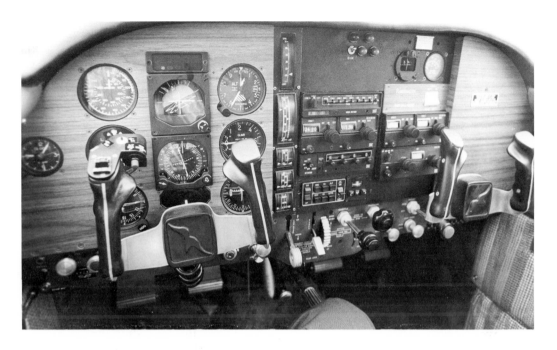

Figure 5-24
illustrates the old primary and supporting power, pitch, and bank instruments. These vary from airplane to airplane, and our purpose here is not to teach you how to fly. Our purpose here is to remind you to believe. Instruments are in the plane for visual reference. Before you believe the seat of your pants or the sensations from your inner ears—believe your eyes.

your vestibular organs. That is, there is now no change in acceleration even though the airplane is still spinning or spiraling. If you then recognize this dilemma and take appropriate corrective movements, you will cause the fluid in your inner ear to create the illusion of spinning in the opposite direction and you will then proceed—if you are dumb enough to believe your vestibular organs—to kick the airplane into a spin in its original direction. The moral, once again, is to believe your gauges and not your ears.

The most dangerous vestibular illusion is the Coriolis illusion, the mechanism of which has already been in part discussed. You will recall that the Coriolis effect is elicited by causing one of the semicircular canals to be suddenly stimulated after the other semicircular canal has already been stimulated and is now in equilibrium. The reason why the Coriolis illusion is most dangerous is that it frequently occurs at critical times when overcorrection can be disastrous. For example, you are over the outer marker in a holding pattern (20 seconds into the final leg turn) and your controller advises you of a change requiring a new approach plate. With your great wisdom, you have the approach plate resting comfortably between your feet. Remember you are still 20 seconds into that turn and your canals have equilibrated. You look down between your feet, bend down and grab your approach plate. You look up suddenly and—bango. Coriolis hits you. The airplane, you, your approach plate, and everything appear upside-down and inside-out. No matter how experienced the pilot, the Coriolis effect can be disastrous. And, if you have been holding at the outer marker under 2,000 feet above ground level, the time needed for recovery might not be adequate. For the third time, the moral is latch onto the gauges fast and believe them.

An illusion caused by our utricle-saccule system is the oculogravic illusion. This is a combined eye-vestibular sense misinteraction. The problem is easy to understand. Our otolith organs are designed for a land environment. Gravity, of course, points down toward the earth. If we accelerate an airplane, a force pushing straight backward is compounded by a gravity force, say at 45 degrees between the horizontal and the vertical. The pilot is suckered into thinking "up" is the direction opposite to that 45-degree vector and therefore thinks that his nose should be 45 degrees down from straight and level. If you believe the illusion created by the otoliths, you then fly the airplane into the ground.

A reverse illusion occurs when you decelerate suddenly. For example, let us say it is night and you are in a tight landing pattern. You throw down your gear and flaps. The deceleration creates the opposite of the illusion just discussed. You think your horizon is 45 degrees down from where it really is and correct rapidly by pulling up. You stall. Most embarrassing! The message once again is rather clear—believe your gauges!

Medical Conditions

Chronic conditions affecting the vestibular apparatus are disqualifying for the flight physical. So it is unlikely that, unless you have a waiver, you will be flying with any vestibular disorder. That is not to say that you cannot be a successful pilot and overcome a vestibular dysfunction. After all, one of our early astronauts underwent surgery for a vestibular disorder called Meniere's disease and was placed in the most compromising of circumstances with no ill effects. That notwithstanding, you should not fly with a known vestibular disorder until you have had appropriate evaluation with electronystagmography and have an appropriate waiver.

There is, however, a situation that can develop and seriously compromises your vestibular function. We are back to that old problem of middle-ear aeration. Recall in our discussion of the middle ear that flying with any sort of eustachian tube blockage (e.g., a cold) is a set-up for a negative middle ear pressure as you descend. This negative pressure can be transmitted to the inner ear fluids, through the round window in the middle ear. When this happens, the vestibular function can be compromised and/or instant vertigo can result. Furthermore, as noted in the ear section, the membrane to the labyrinth can actually rupture, resulting in a sudden loss of fluid pressure in the semicircular canals and

Figure 5-25
is a photograph of a Flightmatic
spatial disorientation trainer. In a
closed environment, the pilot has
cockpit control similar to that of an
airplane. Almost all vestibular illusions can be recreated by this trainer.
Exposure to the trainer is available
at many Air Force flight chamber
installations; the $5 paid to the FAA
for an orientation in one is an
excellent investment.

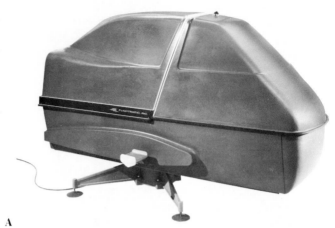

A

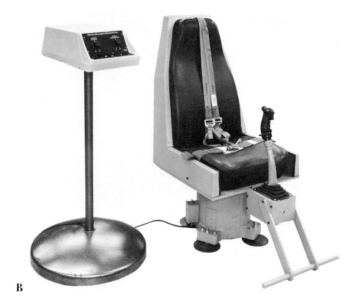

B

instant incapacitating vertigo. The message
should be clear: do not fly when you are sick!

Overview

Vestibular disorientation is worsened by stress-
provoking situations, by hypoxia, by medications

such as cold preparations, and by emotional problems. Disorientation is more common at night, in bad weather conditions and rapidly changing lighting situations, and in inexperienced pilots. Statistics are difficult to compile, but studies have shown that virtually all pilot trainees are subject to vertigo. Approximately one-half end up motion sick. Even among experienced pilots, 25 percent of fatal accidents are presumed caused by spatial disorientation. Of course, less experienced pilots are more prone to spatial disorientation. And the higher performance the craft, the more subject the pilot to spatial disorientation.

How, then, can we prevent spatial disorientation?

First, we must be aware of it. To this end, we have spent a great deal of time in threading our way through a confusing maze of anatomy, physiology, and circuitous explanations. If nothing else, the message must be that spatial disorientation exists and can be incapacitating.

Second, train for disorientation. There is no substitute for having recovered from a host of unusual attitudes under appropriate instruction. Once you have convinced yourself that you can overcome virtually any unusual attitude in which the airplane is placed, you are one more step on the way toward making yourself a safe pilot when disorientation occurs (see Figure 5-25).

Finally, be instrument proficient. The bottom line is believing your eyes. If you can't use your eyes and align the gauges or horizon, all else is to no avail.

CHAPTER 6

ACCIDENTS AND INVESTIGATIONS

Flying is incredibly safe. In spite of over 4,619,900,000 general-aviation miles flown in 1977, there were only 4,476 accidents, 693 resulting in fatalities. Stated in other ways, the fatality rate was only 3.67 per 100,000 aircraft hours or 0.30 per million aircraft miles (see Figure 6-1). Compare that number of fatalities to the 46,880 highway deaths suffered that year. Flying has got to be a safe pastime.

The National Transportation Safety Board released in 1979 a study of 17,312 accidents involving single-engine, propeller-driven, fixed-wing general-aviation airplanes. Of the over 17,000 accidents, 3,517 were fatal and resulted in 6,941 deaths. Analysis by type of aircraft involved 33 makes and demonstrated that the expected fatal accident rate approximated two per 100,000 hours flown.

Overall, single-engine aircraft accounted for 72 percent of all general-aviation hours flown in the

Figure 6-1.
In view of the hue and cry in 1979 regarding the safety of different types of commercial airliners, look at the data in this figure. The accident rate from one plane to the other is not significantly different. In fact, on any given trip, your chances of survival have been estimated at 33 times greater in an airplane than in an automobile.
(U.S. National Transportation Safety Board and National Safety Council)

1968-78 ACCIDENT RATE FOR CERTIFIED U.S. ROUTE CARRIERS

TYPE PLANE	TOTAL ACCIDENTS PER 100,000 MILES FLOWN	FATAL ACCIDENTS PER 100,000 MILES FLOWN
L-1011	1.14	.19
747	0.98	.07
707	0.61	.10
DC-10	0.61	.10
727	0.46	.05

mid-1970s. However, the single-engine craft accounted for 81 percent of the accidents, 76 percent of the fatal accidents, and 69 percent of the fatalities. Although the reasons for these data are poorly understood, it should be apparent to us that those of us flying single-engine craft are the people most at risk. There is no substitute for thinking safety. If we allow safe planning, safe flight, and sound thinking to permeate our concerns—we should be able to improve these statistics.

Reporting Aircraft Accidents

Should you be one of the few involved in an accident, fatal or not, it is imperative that you understand what you must do and the events that will subsequently transpire.

An aircraft operator is required to notify by telephone, telegraph or through the FAA, the nearest National Transportation Safety Board (NTSB) field office following a fatal accident or an accident in which a serious injury or substantial damage to the aircraft has occurred (see Figure 6-2). The regulations define what is meant by fatal injury, serious injury, and substantial damage:

A fatal injury is an injury resulting in death within seven days of the accident.

CRASH REPORTING CHECKLIST

a. Who is reporting the crash? Name, address_____
b. Phone number_____
c. Description of aircraft (type, if known)_____
d. Location of crash_____
e. Directions from nearest town_____
f. Description of crash_____
g. Was fire involved?_____
h. Casualties/ejection seat observed_____
i. Has medical assistance arrived (if necessary)?_____
j. Where will individual meet crash response vehicle to guide party
    to the scene?_____

Figure 6-2
shows the information reporting individuals should give when reporting an aircraft crash.

A serious injury is an injury that requires hospitalization for more than 48 hours within seven days of the accident or results in a fracture of a major bone, a serious laceration and/or hemorrhage, internal-organ injury, or severe burns involving more than five percent of the body surface.

Substantial damage means damage that significantly affects structural strength, performance, or flight characteristics of the airplane. Substantial damage refers to damage requiring a major repair.

Above and beyond the verbal report by telephone, telegraph, or through the FAA, a written report is required within ten days of the accident. Necessary forms can be obtained from NTSB field offices listed in Appendix 8, or through the FAA from their General Aviation District Office (GADOS, see Appendix 9). Part 830 of the FARs, governing rules pertaining to notification and reporting of aircraft accidents, are listed in Appendix 10, with the hope that you will never need them.

Let's assume the worst. If there is an aviation accident involving a fatality, what happens? Most likely the local police will be the first on the scene. The legal responsibility for determining the cause of civil aircraft accidents rests in the hands of the NTSB, which has delegated certain authorities to the FAA. Under the Federal Aviation Act of 1958, the FAA participates with the NTSB to investigate most accidents of fixed-wing aircraft under 12,500 pounds. Thus the NTSB is usually involved in air-carrier or transport fatalities. The FAA is the agency usually responsible for the majority of general-aviation accident investigations, including agriculture and helicopter accidents. When the GADO learns of an accident, it gets on the telephone to the nearest AME and requests that he conduct the medical portion of the accident investigation. The AME is responsible for filing FAA Form 3550, part of which is reproduced as Figure 6-4 on pp. 172-173.

Responsibilities of the AME

The AME is responsible for the aeromedical factors investigation. We are interested in knowing if pilot incapacitation preceded the accident. If human failure was the actual or contributing cause of the accident, items such as myocardial infarction, cerebral vascular accident, major illnesses, carbon monoxide or chemical intoxication, hypoxia, alcohol intoxication, fatigue, and medication all may be involved. The AME is interested in the human factor that might predispose to pilot error, such as the mislocation of an instrument; and he is interested in studying any human failure that can be elicited based on the personal history of the pilot, autopsy or toxicological studies. The AME is responsible for establishing the time of death and determining the relationship between the crash and the injury. He assists in locating and identifying the victims and applies special biomedical techniques to determine the effects of explosives and chemicals, and whether whatever burns he finds occurred before or after death.

The AME brings an accident investigation kit from CAMI (Civil Aeromedical Institute, see Figure 6-3). The basic equipment allows the collection and labeling of specimens (blood, fluid, urine, tissue), their preservation, and transportation. Military kits also include a camera, color film, and flash equipment. The AME usually arranges for a forensic pathologist (medical detective) to perform an autopsy. Prior to removal of the bodies or at time of autopsy, specimens are taken and sent for carbon monoxide levels, alcohol levels, drug levels, and lactic acid levels. It is amazing what the spectrophotometric analysis can detect in blood and tissue. Medications such as barbiturates, tranquilizers, antihistamines, and amphetamines are readily detected. A word to the wise.

If an autopsy is requested by the NTSB representative, then Federal Law mandates its approval. Public Law #87-8010 is applicable to autopsies in fatal aircraft accidents and is stated as follows:

> In carrying out its duties under this title, the Board is authorized to examine and test to the extent necessary any civil aircraft, aircraft engine, propeller, appliance, or property aboard on an aircraft involved in an accident in air commerce. In the case of any fatal accident, the Board is authorized to examine the remains of any deceased person aboard the aircraft at the time of the accident, who dies as a result of the accident, and to conduct autopsies or such other tests thereof as may be necessary to the investigation of the accident: Provided, that to the extent consistent with the needs of the accident investigation, provisions of local law protecting religious beliefs with respect to autopsies shall be observed.

Figure 6-3
is an example of a crash kit used by AMEs for investigating fatal aircraft crashes.
(Courtesy 104th Tactical Clinic and Dr. John J. Cahill)

AVIATION MEDICAL EXAMINERS AIRCRAFT ACCIDENT REPORT	REPORTS IDENTIFICATION SYMBOL

AVIATION MEDICAL EXAMINERS AIRCRAFT ACCIDENT REPORT

Use one Form for each person involved in a fatal accident. For instructions on completion of Form, see handbook AMP 9220.1

REPORTS IDENTIFICATION SYMBOL

AM 9220-2

1. DATE OF ACCIDENT	2. NAME OF VICTIM *(Last - First - Middle Initial)*	VICTIM WAS ☐ PASSENGER ☐ PILOT ☐ OTHER	3. DATE OF BIRTH *(Day, month, year)*
4. AIRCRAFT REGISTRATION NO. **N-**	5. CITY, COUNTY, OR STATE		6. SEAT OCCUPIED

7.		ACCIDENT SITE	8.			TOXICOLOGY	
YES	NO	ITEMS	YES	NO	A. SPECIMEN SUBMITTED FOR	B. NAME AND LOCATION OF LABORATORY	
		A. VISITED			ALCOHOL	
		B. PICTURES TAKEN			CO	
		C. BODY EXAMINED			LACTIC ACID	
		AT SCENE	OTHER *(Specify)*			
		AT MORGUE			C. DRUGS/ALCOHOL FOUND AT SCENE?	
		D. BODY PICTURES TAKEN			☐ YES ☐ NO *(If "Yes," Explain in remarks)*	

9.		AUTOPSY				10.		FIRE	
YES	NO	ITEMS	YES	NO	ITEMS	YES	NO	ITEMS	ESTIMATE (%)
		REQUESTED			X-RAYS TAKEN			AT SCENE	1ST. & 2ND. DEGREE
		OBTAINED			PUBLIC LAW 87-810 USED			BODY BURNED	3RD. DEGREE
If autopsy not obtained, please explain in remarks									INCINERATION

11. REMARKS

FAA Form 3550 (5-64)   (9220)

Figure 6-4.
Sample of Aviation Medical Examiners Aircraft Accident Report.

12.			SAFETY EQUIPMENT	13. DID SEAT DETACH FROM FLOOR?	14. DID VICTIM REMAIN IN THE AIRCRAFT?
YES	NO	UNK.	SEAT BELTS	[ ] YES [ ] NO [ ] UNKNOWN	
			AVAILABLE	IF YES, WAS DETACHMENT	
			USED	[ ] PARTIAL [ ] COMPLETE	[ ] YES [ ] NO
			FAILED		
			SHOULDER HARNESS	DID SEAT SUPPORTS, (Legs) COLLAPSE?	15. OXYGEN EQUIP- MENT AVAILABLE
			AVAILABLE		
			USED	[ ] YES [ ] NO [ ] UNKNOWN	[ ] YES [ ] NO
			FAILED		

CRASH INJURY CORRELATION

16. A crash injury correlation should be done whenever possible, especially in survivable "Accidents." (See page 13). It consists of a gross description of obvious injuries. It is very important to relate aircraft structure to injury area when possible. Below, match the body area with gross injury produced and fill in the square with the Aircraft Structure (Number) which produced the injury.

1. WINDSHIELD
2. CONTROL STICK/WHEEL
3. CONTROL COLUMN
4. INSTRUMENT PANEL
5. STRUCTURE UNDER INSTRUMENT PANEL
6. THROTTLE QUADRANT
7. RUDDER PEDAL
8. SEAT BACK
9. ARM REST

10. SEAT BELT
11. OTHER PERSON
12. AIRCRAFT STRUCTURE OVERHEAD
13. AIRCRAFT STRUCTURE LATERALLY
14. OTHER (Specify)
15. OTHER (Specify)
16. OTHER (Specify)
17. UNKNOWN STRUCTURE
18. BURN, (Any degree)

ITEMS	CONTUSIONS BRUISES	LACERATION	PENETRATION WOUND	OBVIOUS FRACTURE	CRUSHING INJURY	AMPUTATION	EVISCERATING WOUND	BURN
SCALP								
SKULL (Nonfacial)								
FACIAL AREA								
NECK								
THORAX								
ABDOMEN								
PELVIS								
RT. UPPER EXTREMITY								
LEFT UPPER EXTREMITY								
RT. LOWER EXTREMITY								
LEFT LOWER EXTREMITY								

17. NUMBER OF HOURS ON INVESTIGATION BY AVIATION MEDICAL EXAMINER ⟶ HOURS

REQUEST ADDITIONAL COPIES OF FAA FORM 3550 FROM YOUR REGIONAL FLIGHT SURGEON

Figure 6-4 (continued).

It is worth pointing out that the AME participates in the accident investigation as a service to you; he is not compensated for his time.

Protocol

Medical investigation of an aircraft accident for both survivors and fatalities involves five areas: 1. a flying history; 2. a personal history; 3. the human factors investigation; 4. an engineering factors investigation; and 5. laboratory tests and specimens.

Flying history deals with the competence of the pilot based on his training. Is he instrument or commercial rated? Is his biennial certification updated? What extra courses such as the AOPA Safety Courses has he attended? We are most concerned to see if the pilot has had any physiological training in one of the additional FAA or USAF courses. We are concerned with his medical condition to see whether or not he is awaiting admission to a hospital, suffering or convalescing from a disease, or whether or not he has taken any medication recently. Has he suffered from a head injury or heart attack or is he flying with a waiver? We are also interested in his total flying time and the flying time he has in the type of aircraft involved in the accident. We want to know how much time he has flown recently and whether or not his flying has been assessed by other observers.

Personal history is the concern for the pilot's age, marital status, and condition of his or her spouse and/or siblings. We want to know whether he consumes alcohol or tobacco, and what his hobbies or recreational interests are. It is helpful to know the type of car the pilot drives and the condition of its exhaust system. Financial status of the pilot and any eccentricities he might have are important. A previous accident history involving either aircraft, motor vehicles, or third parties is of particular interest. A fatigue history is critical. The time the pilot has been at the controls during this flight, the number of times he has flown recently, the hours of sleep he has received during the last 24 hours and during the last week, and any activities in which he has been involved during the past several days—all are important. In addition, it is important to know the experience time a pilot has had with his present fixed-base operation and how far away from the airfield he lives and has driven.

Human factor addresses physiological stresses, psychological factors, and nutritional status. Physiological stresses include hypoxia, disorientation, heat and cold stress, carbon monoxide intoxication, decompression sickness, incapacitation, hypoglycemia, hyperventilation, and combined stresses such as alcohol, fatigue, and self-medication. Psychological evaluation includes the previous month with regard to the patient's family, personal life, financial and occupational conditions. Life-style factors such as the pilot's habits and activities are important. His general intelligence and emotional stability, his personal characteristics and behavior—all can contribute to an accident. Finally, the nutritional status of the pilot prior to the accident is important. It is valuable to know when the pilot's last meal was eaten, how many hours it was since his last meal, and the composition of his last meal. The pilot's eating habits and whether or not his fluid intake has been adequate are all contributing factors.

Human engineering factors relate to the displays in the cockpit and whether or not they might have been difficult to read or inoperative under the circumstances of the accident. Control switches should be checked to see if they were difficult to reach, impossible to move, or had inadvertently been activated. Finally, if oxygen has been required, examination of the life-support equipment from the oxygen mask to the container itself is critical. A human engineering investigation of the accident equipment is the ultimate PRICE check. Finally, the FAA is interested to know if the location or design of a switch or cockpit enclosure contributed to body trauma.

Lab tests will involve removal of at least six 10 cc tubes of blood and a 50 cc urine specimen. These will be collected to analyze for carbon monoxide, alcohol, sugar, drugs, hemoglobin concentration, and lactic acid. If a fatality is involved, tissue, including a sample of the heart, lungs, and kidneys will also be sent for analysis (see Figure 6-4).

All of the above considerations are taken into account by your AME during an accident investigation. Your job, as an aircraft commander or passenger, is to cooperate. The findings must, of course, be reported on Form 3550 and submitted to the FAA and thence to the National Transportation Safety Board.

Types and Causes of Accidents

Accidents are divided into vertical and horizontal types. The vertical type of accident (see Figure 6-5) is one in which from a significant altitude the airplane progresses out of control into the

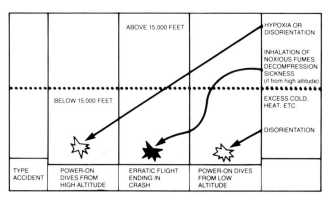

Figure 6-5
demonstrates one of two broad categories of accidents—a vertical type accident. Vertical types tend to be associated with disorientation, climatic conditions, incapacitation, and physical causes at high altitudes. The type of accident frequently gives a clue to the cause.

ground. This type of accident has the highest incidence of fatality. A horizontal-type accident results from a smaller angle of ground impact (see Figure 6-6). Horizontal accidents present a better chance for survival.

Cause

Safely, and without trepidation, we can say that almost all accidents are a result of pilot deficiencies. When considering all causal factors, less than 10 percent of accidents are caused by equipment malfunction. Observation of Appendix 11 immediately reveals that equipment malfunction is most often related to gear and/or tire failure.

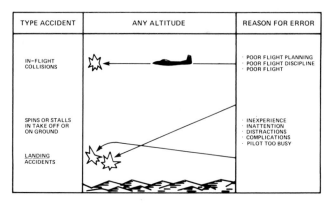

Figure 6-6
demonstrates the horizontal accident.

A disturbing facet of the population of pilots involved in accidents that are nonfatal is the number of pilots who are frequent repeaters and who sometimes ultimately end up on the fatality list. One cannot help but question what makes these accident-prone pilots accident-prone. The signposts seem to hang out from every cloud to all but the pilots involved. Perhaps if you, as a pilot involved in an accident, are reading this, you should ask yourself this question: Am I accident-prone? For those of us involved and those of us with friends involved, extra care for the pilot with an accident record is a must.

Unsafe Pilot Actions

Unsafe pilot actions can be divided into six categories: 1. capacity deficiencies; 2. inadequate knowledge or experience; 3. application deficiencies; 4. attitude deficiencies; 5. deficiencies in aids to flying; and 6. complications and distractions.

Capacity deficiencies include those deficiencies of physical strength, stamina, and ability as well as deficiencies in intelligence and emotional stability. Because of our careful AME medical screening program, capacity deficiencies are rare causes of accidents.

Inadequate knowledge or experience is a significant cause of accidents. Transitioning into new or different airplanes, failure to maintain currency in flying proficiency, and experiencing emergency procedures all can account for an unsafe act and subsequent accident.

Application deficiencies are characterized by

inadequate concentration such as in shooting an instrument approach. Failure to consider hazards such as thunderstorms can also be classified as an application deficiency.

Attitude deficiencies are found in those pilots who have a negative attitude toward flying regulations, who do not obey the rules, and who just do not have the proper mental attitudes for safe flight.

Deficiencies in aids to flying occur when the pilot is too dependent on the multitude of aids that tell him how his airplane is functioning and where he is relative to the ground. Failure of structure or instrumentation can cause an accident, although this is rare.

Complications and distractions, finally, are those factors, such as a sudden downdraft on final, that can account for an accident even when all five of the above deficiencies are not contributory.

Education about high accident risk times is important in helping us be more aware of periods during which we will be at maximum hazard. A good source is Dan Manningham's book *Staying Current.* The facts are elucidated there in very readable fashion to alert us to high risk periods. For example, we find that 50 percent of accidents are on or around an airport. When we are near an airport we should pay the closest attention to all the rules of flying. Night accidents occur with disproportionally high frequency. Perhaps some of this is due to optical illusions created by the pilot; however, maximum attention is demanded during this interval. We know that the most critical instrument approach in terms of a disproportionate accident rate is a circling approach. Perhaps we should raise our minima. Finally, we learn that the attitude of the pilot is the bottom line in accident prevention. The pilot with a positive attitude will seek out information regarding accidents so that for him history will not repeat itself.

Accident Research

There are approximately 4,000 light plane accidents per year. Recognition of the fact that a certain number of people perish in these accidents has led to a research program currently being directed by NASA toward general-aviation aircraft. One study demonstrated that fully two-thirds of pilots and passengers killed suffered fatal skull fractures while half had received severe spinal injuries; both of these findings suggest better crash survivability if documentation of those factors responsible for the injuries can be obtained.

As of this writing, 21 crash simulations by NASA researchers have been enacted. A variety of planes, many donated by Piper Aircraft, had been crashed from a 240-foot-high, 400-foot-long test gantry. Research was conducted in much the same way as in automobile crash studies. Lines were painted along the fuselage to demonstrate deformation characteristics for the cameras. The airplanes were loaded with G meters, dummies with electrodes connected, and a variety of restraint systems. A pattern of problems is evolving from this research that allows the occupants to sustain injuries above and beyond what might be expected if further safeguards were taken. It was found that seats frequently separate from their tracks and hurl the occupants into the dashboard. It was found that seats firmly attached over a spar structure do not deform and thus transmit impacts to the occupants more readily. It was found that a double shoulder harness anchored to a firm seat or to the main airplane structure is the most effective restraining device. It was found that the nine-G requirement for seat attachments must be increased to 20 or 30 Gs to save more lives. It was found that fewer projections from the instrument panel and a padded instrument panel lead to better crash survivability.

Although these tests are ongoing and conclusions are at this time indefinite, it seems likely that data obtained from these tests will lead to a basis for different regulations for our general aviation manufacturers, which may very well increase the pilot and passenger ability to survive an accident (see Figure 6-7 on pp. 182-183).

OVERVIEW

Aircraft accidents are, of course, extremely rare. When considering accidents in this chapter, we are confining our observations to major accidents in contradistinction to minor accidents. Accident rates vary from year to year, but have most recently been reported as approximately four fatalities per 100,000 flying hours. The effect of the accident, of course, can result in loss of life, economic loss, and bad public relations for all of us in flying. In fact, passenger fatalities per 100,000,000 passenger miles are approximately threefold in autos as compared with domestic scheduled airlines. All in all, we do really well, but we must keep bringing the message to our doubting public. With approximately 70 million flights per year, there have been only about 650 airplane crashes per year, which in 1978 resulted

IDENTIFICATION STRIP: *Please fill in all blanks. This section will be returned to you promptly; no record will be kept.*

TELEPHONE NUMBERS where we may reach you
for further details of this occurrence:

AREA _____ NO. _____ HOURS _____

AREA _____ NO. _____ HOURS _____

NAME _____

ADDRESS _____

TYPE OF OCCURRENCE/INCIDENT: _____

DATE OF OCCURRENCE _____

TIME *(local, 24-hr. clock)* _____

(This space reserved for NASA
time receipt stamp)

Except for reports of accidents and criminal activities, all identities contained in this report will
be removed to assure complete reporter confidentiality.

Please fill in appropriate spaces and circle or check all terms which apply to this occurrence or incident.

1. Location: *(Geographic (including State), airport, runway, ATC facility and sector, navigation aid reference, etc.)*

2. Type of operation:

SCHEDULED AIR CARRIER	SUPPLEMENTAL CARRIER	CORPORATE AVIATION	MILITARY ARMY
DOMESTIC OPERATION	CHARTER OPERATION	PERSONAL BUSINESS	NAVY CG MC
INTERNATIONAL OPN	UTILITY OPERATION	PLEASURE FLIGHT	AIR FORCE
AIR TAXI	AGRICULTURAL OPN	TRAINING FLIGHT	GOVERNMENT

3. Type of aircraft:

FIXED WING, LOW	RETRACTABLE GEAR	RECIPROCATING	GROSS WT <2500	25,000-50,000
HIGH WING	CONST SPEED PROP	TURBOPROP	2500-5000	50,000-100,000
ROTARY WING	FLAPS	TURBOJET	5000-12,500	100,000-300,000
NO OF SEATS	NO OF ENGINES	WIDE BODY JET	12,500-25,000	OVER 300,000

4. Second aircraft TYPE: *(if two aircraft involved)*

5. Reported by: PILOT   CREWMEMBER   CONTROLLER   OTHER *(specify)*

   If pilot: **TOTAL HOURS:**   **HRS. LAST 90 DAYS:**

6. Light conditions: DAWN   DAYLIGHT   DUSK   NIGHT   7. Altitude: _____ FEET MSL.

| 8. Flight plan: | IFR | VFR | DVFR | SVFR | NONE | | 9. Flight conditions: | VFR | IFR |

10. Flight phase: PREFLIGHT TAXI TAKEOFF CLIMB CRUISE DESCENT
HOLDING TRAFFIC PATTERN APPROACH LANDING MISSED APPROACH

11. Airspace: POSITIVE CONTROL AREA (PCA) TERMINAL CONTROL AREA (TCA) ON AIRWAYS
AIRPORT TRAFFIC AREA UNCONTROLLED AIRSPACE OTHER CONTROLLED AIRSPACE

12. Air Traffic Control: GROUND TOWER DEPARTURE CENTER APPROACH FSS NONE

13. Weather factors: RESTRICTED VISIBILITY TURBULENCE THUNDERSTORM AIRCRAFT ICING
CROSSWIND PRECIPITATION NONE OTHER (specify)

14.
(Circle all which you believe apply to this occurrence)

AIRPORT AIR TRAFFIC CONTROL AIR NAVIGATION FACILITY AIRCRAFT
FLIGHT CREW AERONAUTICAL PUBLICATION/CHARTS OTHER (specify below)

15. NARRATIVE DESCRIPTION: Please describe the occurrence as clearly and precisely as possible. Include information on: what happened . . . how was the problem discovered . . . what actions were taken . . . was evasive action required . . . what factors contributed to the situation . . . why do you believe the situation occurred . . . your suggestions as to how to prevent a recurrence.
USE BOTH SIDES OF THE FORM, AS REQUIRED.

Continue on other side.

Figure 6-7.
In late summer of 1979, the FAA appointed the National Aeronautics and Space Administration as an independent evaluating agency for the Aviation Safety Reporting Program (ASRP). Thus, any reports turned in to NASA will not be held against the pilot by the FAA. The reporting form and portions of the advisory are reproduced here in the hope that pilots will take advantage of the opportunity to report any unsafe conditions. Only through this type of reporting can we direct education and rehabilitation to initiate appropriate action.

183

in 1,709 deaths. This compares most favorably with the over 50,000 1978 highway deaths. In spite of the fear on the part of many passengers, there have been only 50 airline collisions in over 40 years of flying, proving that flying is an incredibly safe form of transportation.

CHAPTER 7

The Medical Preflight

FOUR AREAS of CONCERN

Happy flying depends on satisfying four areas of concern: having a current medical certificate, having gone over a medical preflight checklist, having appropriate medical equipment on board, and having appropriate survival gear on board.

Current medical certification. Chapter 1 outlines the requirements and limitations of your medical certification. Remember that a Class III physical—the one required for most general aviation pilots—is currently valid for two years following the last day of the month in which you obtained the physical. If you do not have a valid medical certificate, stay out of the air until you have seen an AME.

Medical preflight checklist. A medical preflight checklist is as important as an aircraft checklist. Unless you are fit and tuned in to potential medical problems, you should not be cranking up. Recall the physiological stresses

MEDICAL EQUIPMENT PREFLIGHT

1. Nose spray for ear and sinus blocks
2. Handkerchief
3. Motion sickness bag
4. Clothing for above and on the ground survival
5. Survival gear:
    1. Raft if over water
    2. Flares
    3. Radio

**Figure 7-1
is a list of basic flight medical
equipment. This equipment is no
less important than carrying appropriate records and survival gear in
your airplane.**

discussed in Chapters 2 and 3. Remember that a tired pilot is an accident-prone pilot. Remember hypoxia. Use oxygen equipment; use the PRICE check. If you smoke, remember to use oxygen from the ground up at night. Smoker or not, always use oxygen from 10,000 feet and up. Avoid dehydration. Remember that water loading is not required; take along a thermos of water and sip as you go. Be prepared for disorientation; remember that the white portion of the attitude gyro belongs on top. We are all subject to disorientation, and all of us will experience disorientation at some time during our flying career. Maximize your circadian rhythms to fly at your peak times. If traveling, obtain adequate rest to compensate for changes in circadian rhythm.

Psychological stress can be as incapacitating as a physical malady. Emotion belongs on the ground and not in the air.

Medication while flying is a no-no. If congested on descent, use the local nasal spray in the medical equipment kit. If you have any questions about flying with medication, consult your AME.

You have no business flying without eating first because food is energy. Don't raise blood sugar rapidly and then lower it rapidly by eating junk food prior to flight. Remember to avoid gas-producing carbonated beverages.

Sleep and exercise are important in maintaining a healthy pilot's body. A person who is physically fit is bound to be more precise and capable as a pilot and will be able to withstand both the physical and mental stresses of flying.

Alcohol has no place in a flying environment. The rule of eight hours from bottle to throttle is a bare minimum.

Immunizations within the United States are accomplished as part of routine school innocula-tions. Should you travel outside of the United

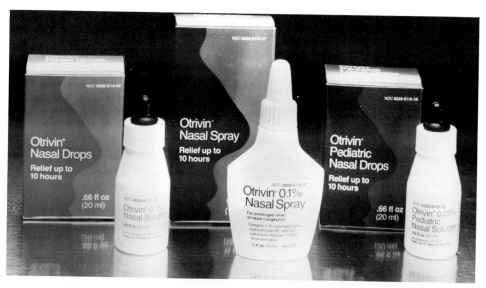

States, then you should give some thought to the endemic diseases of the areas into which you are entering. Immunizations are further discussed in this chapter.

Finally, area health hazards should be anticipated. Such hazards range from a cold climate to water, and from desert to snake bites. Think out the area over which you are flying and the area in which you will arrive to anticipate problems before you face them.

Medical Equipment Preflight. A medical supply inventory is simple and should be part of your routine flight procedures. Most pilots carry a flight case, containing the AIM, instrument approach plates, three-cell flashlight, gas credit cards, kneeboard, flight computer, FAA license, physical certificate, radio permit, pencil and paper, and some extra cash. I carry all of the foregoing equipment in my flight case, which sits in the trunk of my car and is part of every flight I take—short or long. In addition, I also carry in that case all of the medical equipment listed in Figure 7-1: a bottle of Otrivin for ear or sinus blocks (see Figure 7-2), a handkerchief, two

Figure 7-2.
Part of every flight kit should be a spray container of a long-acting nasal decongestant medication such as Otrivin. Since one never knows when a sinus or ear block can occur, you must carry a local decongestant medication that will provide for relief of sinus and/or ear symptoms, both of which can lead to incapacitating pain or vertigo. A long-acting nasal spray such as Otrivin should be employed after reascending, should an ear or sinus block occur. Otrivin is available from your local FAA medical examiner as a prescription medication. Its shelf life is long, and it can be carried in your flight case for many months.
(Courtesy Geigy Pharmaceuticals)

SUGGESTED SURVIVAL KIT CONTENTS

1. Life raft or flotation gear
2. Survival radio with spare battery
3. Signal mirror
4. Distress signal (flare)
5. Waterproof matches
6. Drinking water in sealed container with appropriate opener
7. Whistle
8. First-aid kit
9. Life raft repair kit
10. Marker dye
11. Plastic bag (one gallon)
12. Jackknife
13. Blanket
14. Emergency rations
15. Wool socks
16. Brass wire (20-foot coil)
17. Snake-bite kit
18. Long-burning candle
19. Winter hood
20. Survival manual (see Appendix 12)
21. Aluminum foil
22. Towelettes (six)
23. Leather mittens with wool inserts

Figure 7-3.
The 23 items listed here form a basic survival kit. Additions to these basics will vary, depending on the type of terrain over which you fly.

motion-sickness bags, wool gloves, a wool pull-over hat, and a nylon survival jacket in bright orange are all part of the kit. I also carry a penetrating flare gun (Colt) as well as night and day ground flares and an emergency (121.5) locating radio with transmitting capability and a 12-hour battery supply. The only survival equipment I sometimes add is an inflatable raft, if I anticipate over-water travel. The medical equipment check is as much a part of your flying activity as the aircraft preflight.

Surviving the Crash. Having read Chapter 6, "Aircraft Accidents," you are well aware that most of us would survive an aircraft accident if we had appropriate survival gear on board. There should be basic survival gear on board, some of which may be carried in your regular flight case. The 23 items listed in Figure 7-3 compose a survival kit complement. There will be much variation of contents depending on the area over which you will be flying. There is no right or wrong in survival gear. Nonetheless, it is important to think about the geography over which you will be flying and to give some thought to those items that could be life-saving. In our medical equipment checklist, we have already alluded to a survival radio and flares. Why not add a few little goodies that are not space or weight consuming, such as a signal

Figure 7-4.
Nicolet Products produces a packaged survival kit that satisfies most needs. The kit is available through most aviation supply houses and/or your fixed-base operator.

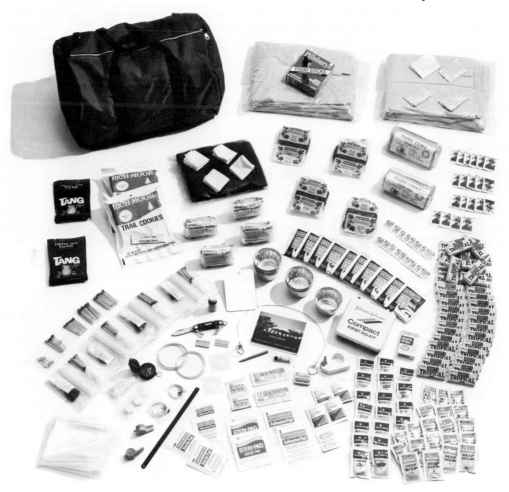

CONSIDERATIONS FOR HELICOPTER TRANSPORT

1. Time: Can helicopter provide faster transport than ground ambulance?
2. Patient Pickup Site: Is suitable helicopter landing site available?
3. Severity of Injury: Air transport indicated to prevent death or aggravation of the illness or injury of the patient?
4. Resource Availability: Is ground transport, appropriate medical personnel and significant medical equipment available?

MASSACHUSETTS MAST COMMITTEE
(413) 557-2941
MILITARY ASSISTANCE TO SAFETY & TRAFFIC

ADMINISTRATIVE:
1. Requestor Name and Service.
2. Location, Street, Town, Geographical Landmarks.
3. Requestor's Radio Frequency.
4. Landing Area and any Restrictions.
5. Landing Site Identification.
6. Destination of Patient.

MEDICAL:
7. Number of Patients (litter) (ambulatory).
8. Condition of Patient: Injury, Age, Sex.
9. Specialized Equipment Needed.

Figure 7-5.
The first responders to an air evacuation emergency are usually emergency medical technicians (EMTs) working for police or fire departments or ambulance companies. These responders usually carry a wallet-size card, such as that shown here, that provides the vital information needed for arranging a helicopter pick-up.

mirror, a whistle, a jackknife, a small can of rations, and waterproof matches? Take a good look at Figures 7-3 and 7-4. Give some thought to how you would survive in the wilderness until a search party finds you. If you have enough equipment on board to satisfy your needs, you have done your job. If not, you should learn to think *safety*. Thinking safety is thinking survival by anticipating the worst. My survival kit is prewrapped exclusive of those items in my flight case, which require routine maintenance. I leave my survival kit packed in the airplane. The only item I add is a life raft, when one is required.

EVACUATION

Many areas in which crashes occur are inaccessible with conventional means of transportation. To fill the need for medical evacuation in areas to

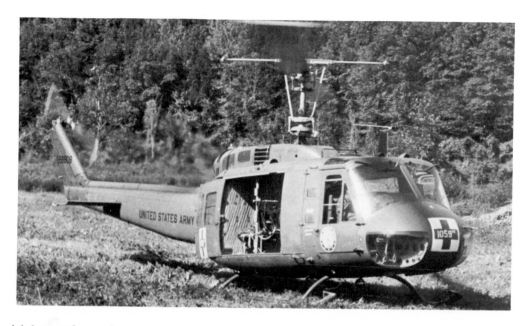

which roads and/or ambulance service is not readily available, the MAST Program was created. MAST is an acronym for Military Assistance to Safety and Traffic Program, which originated in July of 1970. An interagency executive group with representatives from the U.S. Departments of Transportation, Defense, and Health and Human Services created the MAST Program. MAST serves to supplement existing civilian emergency programs and assist local communities, state police, fire departments, and emergency medical corporations (see Figure 7-5). MAST employs military Medevac helicopters organized to assist in civilian emergencies. MAST serves to transport patients from accident sites to hospitals, between hospitals, and to transport donor organs and biological fluids such as blood (see Figure 7-6).

To a pilot, MAST means evacuation from any area no matter how inaccessible the site might be. If a helicopter cannot land at the site, a hoist can provide evacuation, as was done by rescuers in Vietnam. Patients who are too badly injured to hang onto a hoist themselves will be assisted by a

Figure 7-6.
A UH-1 Medovac Helicopter is routinely employed in MAST missions. This helicopter can lift victims through a 250-foot canopy by way of a hoist. If necessary, a medic can be lowered on the hoist to give assistance. This should provide incentive for pilots to carry an ELT and a portable two-way radio such as is carried in the military. MAST helicopters have the ability to be launched in five minutes from the time of announced emergency and usually service an area within 100 nautical miles of their base.

medic who is lowered with the hoist. As of this writing, there are over 30 MAST units organized throughout the continental United States. The MAST unit has the potential for serving a very valuable function in the rescue of pilots. You should know about it so that you too may request it.

Once the patient has been evacuated to an area where conventional planes can land, a fixed-wing air ambulance is frequently brought in, for it is less expensive and has a greater range as well as speed than does a helicopter. To fill this void, air ambulance companies are being formed throughout the country (see Figure 7-7).

Basic Medical Briefing

Pilots who travel in caravans to attend meetings, vacations, or travel long distances will do well to have a briefing by a local AME prior to departure. Most are happy to spend an evening with a group, to present a slide show and hand

Figure 7-7.
A new area contributing to pilot and passenger safety is the medical evacuation air ambulance. Serious injuries requiring specialized or complicated care can be safely and rapidly transported to an appropriate center. Based on wartime experience in Vietnam, this new air ambulance service should contribute to increased survival of seriously injured accident victims.
(Compliments **Dr. Wesley W. Bare, North American Air Ambulance**)

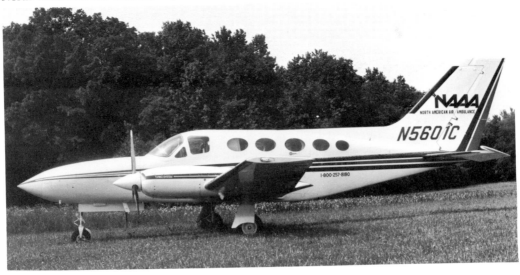

out a printed briefing, to give medical orientation to the problems that may be faced during your trip. Such a discussion places the burden of research on the backs of the AMEs, in order to seek out those problems that are peculiar, medically, to a particular trip. For those of you who do not have such an AME readily available, following is a simple medical briefing.

There are multiple considerations that must be reviewed prior to any flight:

- Special medical matters
- Diet
- Fluid
- Alcoholic beverages
- Rest
- Special medications
- Adequate preflight time
- Special clothing
- Conditions under flight
- In-flight considerations
- Post-flight considerations

Let's look at the meaning of each of these sections.

Special medical matters, pertaining to the area to which you are going to fly, relate primarily to endemic diseases and special environmental considerations. For example, if you are going to be traveling to an area in which there is malaria, an appropriate prophylaxis, as suggested in Figure 7-8 (p. 200), should be considered. The point is to give thought to those matters that are going to require special consideration when you finally arrive. You are further ahead of the game in taking special medication and/or directions for treatment with you than you would be worrying about obtaining the medication and/or the proper treatment after you arrive in an area. You would be well advised to carry a survival kit as noted in Figure 7-4. Add appropriate emergency preparations such as water purification tablets and antidiarrheal medication.

Diet. A high-protein, low-residue diet is your best bet as a pilot or crew member. The old classic steak-and-egg breakfast is a good standby. Try to avoid carbohydrates, which tend to be fatiguing. For insight into the effect of food on your circadian rhythm, take a look at our discussion on page 117 wherein we comment on the use of high-protein and caffeine in initiating a good biological rhythm. Try to avoid very filling, bulk-producing diets, which are going to pose a problem for you in terms of elimination or constipation.

Fluids. Fluid intake should be as normal as possible. Do not overhydrate by drinking an excess amount of fluid on the assumption this will last you longer. You are far better to take a thermos of water than you are loading up before the flight. Thirst is a good guide as to proper fluid replenishment. Remember that increased airflow, and especially higher temperatures, will increase your need for fluid intake. Do not use salt tablets as a means for retaining fluid. Remember that carbonated beverages pose two problems for the pilot: first, they tend to get your attention when opened at 10,000 feet in a non-pressurized environment; and second, they produce gas and increase your chances for dysbarism (see Chapter 2). You are well advised to stick with water and/or coffee. Remember to change your thermos at each landing lest the water get flat and/or rancid.

Alcoholic beverages. The rule of eight hours from bottle to throttle has already been discussed. A much better rule is to avoid any alcoholic beverage for 24 hours prior to flight. As you well know, the effects of alcohol on body systems extend above and beyond the direct chemical toxicity. Dehydration, hypoglycemia, and fatigue are all the result of alcohol ingestion. Alcohol has little or no role in an active pilot's life.

Rest. The military has a requirement that 12 hours of crew rest is required prior to flight. Yet so many of us civilians easily hop into our planes, especially when we are tired. Mental and physical coordination decrease, and mistakes tend to snowball. Rest is as important a part of your physical preflight as is making certain that the plane is in good condition. Make sure to allow eight hours' uninterrupted sleep prior to your rising and still have enough time for adequate flight preparations. A well-rested pilot is a pilot who is free of worries and is physically and mentally prepared to take on any problems that emerge during his flight. Adequate, proper rest is surely underplayed. Remember our circadian rhythm discussion—your body is bound to have peaks with highs and valleys with lows as it progresses through its normal daily cycle. Take advantage of the highs; fly when well rested.

Special medications. Medications to arouse the pilot are not approved by the FAA. But coffee, with its caffeine content, is a legal stimulant. Awake in time to get your act together prior to hopping into the plane. This means that you should get up in time to have an adequate breakfast, with coffee if you need it. Obtain a good weather briefing, file your flight plan, preflight your airplane, get your passengers properly situated and in a relaxed state; crank it up. Don't try to beat the system by using sleeping medication or stimulant pills. First, they are illegal. Second, they don't accomplish what you think; sleeping medication actually deprives you of dream time, which is the prerequisite of a good, restful sleep. Stay with a normal rest–activity cycle and you will stay out of trouble.

Adequate preflight time.   Rising from bed in time to run out to the airplane, make a cursory observation of its mechanical state, jump in, and crank up just doesn't hack it. Adequate preflight time means that you have enough time to get your act together before going out to the plane. This means washing up, a trip to the toilet to relieve yourself, any adequate breakfast to get your body moving, and, finally, a leisurely trip to the hangar. Now is the time to check the weather reports (regardless of what it may look like in the sky), to file a flight plan (regardless of whether or not you are IFR bound), and to make certain that you have gone through the medical briefing checklist. Then, and only then, should you make your trip to the plane, again, with enough time to check out all of its systems thoroughly. There is the story of the young student who was observing an old man walk around his Tri-pacer ten times. The student turned to his flight inspector and chided, "The old man is going to get dizzy looking at that plane." Replied the flight instructor, "Yes, that's Charles Lindbergh. He once said that the only time he had to correct a problem was while he was on the ground and not after he had taken off."

Special clothing.   Protective gear for the flight should be donned prior to your leaving the heated automobile or hangar. There is no point in your arriving in an airplane in a half-frozen state, taking off with numb fingers, and waiting for the perhaps malfunctioning airplane heater to suck in carbon monoxide and warm you up. You must anticipate flying in the environment in which you are walking. Protective gear includes sunglasses. Clothing should be anticipated based on your current climate conditions, the weather conditions that you may or may not anticipate at your destination, and the terrain, or water conditions, over which you are going to be flying.

Conditions under flight. Long before you hop into the left seat, you should have considered the conditions under flight. If you are going to be flying at a comfortable level on the ground, which turns into a freezing level in the sky, dress accordingly. It is naive for you to expect the plane's heating system to be flawless. Adequate preflight considerations provide you with appropriate oxygen supplies for the length of the trip, for all passengers on board, and enough to compensate for your alternate airport or for an in-flight emergency. Conditions under flight also apply to those items that should be carried for passengers and perhaps your comfort. For example, motion-sickness bags should be part of the equipment of every airplane. If you have never been airsick, you haven't flown enough! (See the discussion of motion sickness in Chapter 3.) Think out the trip, anticipate the problems before they occur, and prepare for them while you are still on the ground.

In-flight considerations refer primarily to food, water, and oxygen. We have already taken into consideration adequate clothing, eye protection, and oxygen. Food should be small and easy to handle. If worst comes to worst, you should still be able to handle the controls and eat! Small, bite-size sandwiches, hard candies, and fruit are all good flying food. Remember that under some conditions oxygen masks will have to be removed for short periods of time in order to ingest the foods, so keep your meals rapidly eatable, small, and easily digestible. Remember that it is far better to eat lightly and frequently than to gobble the food all at one time. With regard to fluid, water is still your best bet. Make sure that the water is fresh. Avoid large amounts of coffee since it tends to make you urinate; avoid carbonated beverages because of the problem in handling them in the plane as well as in dealing with their urinary effects. Take along a relief bottle so that you can urinate in flight. Don't confuse the jugs.

Post-flight considerations. Your medical concerns do not stop when you hit the ground. Now is the time to consider any factors that might have an impact on your stay on the ground or on future flights: rest, food, hydration, immunizations, and appropriate prophylactic medication should all be checked meticulously. Treat any problems, such as an ear blockage, which may have arisen during flight. Then have a good stay.

International Travel

If you are thinking of flying outside the United States, you should be aware of health hazards peculiar to the country in which you are traveling. An excellent source to which you may turn is called *Health Information for International Travel.* This U.S. Department of Health and Human Services Centers for Disease Control publication is available from the Bureau of Epidemiology Quarantine Division, Atlanta, Georgia 30333 (HEW Publications #CDC78-8280).

Leafing through the 96 pages of this booklet will reveal vaccination information, vacation certificate requirements, public health recommendations, specific immunotherapy and prophylaxis suggestions, health hints for the traveler, reentry-of-pet information, and importation or exportation of human remains information. These last items are not included to make you nervous about flying outside the country.

For purposes of international health regulations, you should know that the incubation period of the quarantinable diseases are cholera—5 days; plague—6 days; smallpox—14 days; and yellow fever—6 days. There is a weekly "Blue Sheet" distributed to public health officers. If you are worried about the area to which you are planning to travel with regard to potential infection, call the nearest Public Health office and ask them to check their "Blue Sheet."

The World Health Organization has distributed certain international health regulations with regard to certificates of vaccination against cholera, smallpox, and yellow fever. You should know that your certificate is valid for six months following a cholera injection, for three years after your smallpox injection, and for ten years after your yellow fever injection. There are no vaccination requirements for traveling between the United States, Europe, Canada, Mexico, and the Caribbean. There are no vaccinations required for returning to this country. *Health Information for International Travel* lists the requirements of each country individually, taking about 50 pages to do this. In a nutshell, the United States recommends a yellow fever vaccination for travel to infected areas, but beyond this, there are no specific recommendations. However, this recommendation is based on the presumption that all Americans will have been immunized to common

MALARIA PROPHYLAXIS

DOSE	COMMENTS
Chloroquine phosphate 500 mg (300 mg base) orally once a week beginning 1 week prior to arrival, during the stay, and continuing 6 weeks after departure	Infants and children up to 50 kg* in body weight should receive 5 mg (base)/kg body weight. All persons over 50 kg can be given full dose chemoprophylaxis. Pediatric suspension preparations are available commercially in some countries but not in the United States. Pharmacists in the United States may be able to prepare suspensions for pediatric use.

*kg = approximately 2.2 lbs.

Figure 7-8
is the Public Health Service recommended doses schedule for malaria prophylaxis. Remember that antimalarial medication is frequently nauseating. You are well advised to try the medication before you fly.

diseases such as diphtheria, tetanus, pertussis, polio, measles, mumps, and rubella.

Although immunotherapy (a shot) is not available for malaria, our Public Health Service recommends that travelers into known malaria areas take malaria prophylactic drugs. A recommended dose schedule is shown in Figure 7-8.

International airports frequently have a medical facility, which can help in identifying immunizations required for entering foreign countries.

There is a short, 19-page leaflet produced by the American Medical Association called *Physician's Guide to Medical Advice for Overseas Travelers.* It is the AMA's position that, although not required by the World Health Organization, it is advantageous to be immunized to as many common diseases as practicable. For those who have not had the advantage of a disensitization program as a child, or in the service, they offer a rapid immunization program that can be completed in 16 days. This program is as follows:

16-Day Rapid Immunization Program for Adults

First Day	*Typhoid, Tetanus-Diphtheria*
Second Day	*Yellow Fever*
Third Day or Fourth Day	*Influenza*

Fifth Day	*Cholera, Typhus*
Ninth Day	*Typhoid, Smallpox*
Twelfth Day	*Typhus, Cholera, Inspect Smallpox*
Sixteenth Day	*Typhoid, Tetanus-Diphtheria, Gamma Globulin, Inspect Smallpox*

Travelers' Health Hints

Most of us will not know the conditions of a foreign country until we arrive there. Under these circumstances, it behooves us to plan ahead so that we are not caught short. If you wear glasses, take an extra pair or at least your lens prescription. Take along a bracelet or a printed history sheet identifying any physical condition that might require emergency care. If you need a physician when you are in a foreign country, think of a travel agency or the American embassy. Any prescription medications that you carry should be accompanied by a letter from your doctor. You should also include any statement of major health problems that might require emergency care. Try to carry your own drugs when at all possible. Bear in mind that most patients who become ill while traveling in another country do so within six weeks after returning from travel. There are, however, some diseases, such as malaria, which may not show up for as long as six months after you have completed traveling. Therefore, when a physician takes a history from you of any recent foreign travels, make sure to include the past year in your history.

Water

You should always be skeptical of water in a foreign country. Few countries have the standard of chlorination and bacteria counts as a quality control that is present in the United States. Try to drink beverages made from boiled water, such as coffee or tea. Use canned or bottled carbonated beverages. Beer and wine are usually safe (although not for the flier, obviously). Regard ice as being as contaminated as the water from which it is made. Should you have to use the local water, boil the water for ten minutes, then allow the water to cool at room temperature. There are commercial preparations made for making water safe to drink, such as Halazone tablets. You may also purify water with tincture of iodine; add five drops of 2 percent tincture of iodine per quart of water. You may also add laundry bleach (chlorine) to water; two drops per quart of 4 to 6 percent chlorine will do the trick.

Diarrhea

Diarrhea can seem almost inevitable when one is traveling in a foreign country. Even when intestinal infections do not take place, the change of food habits and/or the local normal bacteria result in "the revenge." If you have blood or mucus in your stool and/or fever is present, then you should consult a physician and not try to treat the diarrhea yourself. If you have diarrhea, bear in mind that you will become dehydrated. Salts and fluids are lost—especially potassium. So, you will have to reconstitute yourself with fluids such as carbonated drinks, tea, and even canned fruit juices. If your stomach is not too irritated, tomatoes, bananas, and orange juice do a good job in replenishing the depleted potassium. Baking soda (half a teaspoon) in a glass of water may serve to settle the stomach. It is a good idea to take along an antidiarrhea pill, such as Lomotil, for helping control hyperactive bowels.

EMERGENCY CPR PROCEDURES

I feel strongly that all citizens should be trained in cardiopulmonary resuscitation (CPR). The health and safety of his passengers are the pilot's special responsibility, for he is the commander of the aircraft. These circumstances in themselves mandate that all pilots be familiar with CPR procedures. Figure 7-9 lists the basics for taking care of a catastrophe in the cockpit. This type of card is available from the Government Printing Office and is worth carrying in your flight case.

Figure 7-9 shows emergency procedures for shock victims with which all pilots should be familiar. Although an approved CPR course is advisable, the information in this figure is the next best bet.

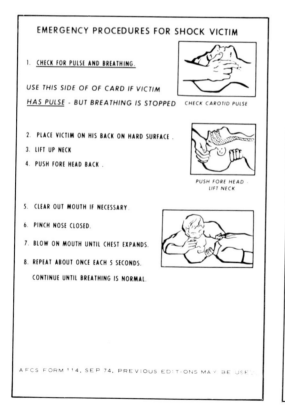

EMERGENCY PROCEDURES FOR SHOCK VICTIM

1. CHECK FOR PULSE AND BREATHING.

USE THIS SIDE OF OF CARD IF VICTIM HAS PULSE - BUT BREATHING IS STOPPED

CHECK CAROTID PULSE

2. PLACE VICTIM ON HIS BACK ON HARD SURFACE.
3. LIFT UP NECK
4. PUSH FORE HEAD BACK.

PUSH FORE HEAD - LIFT NECK

5. CLEAR OUT MOUTH IF NECESSARY.
6. PINCH NOSE CLOSED.
7. BLOW ON MOUTH UNTIL CHEST EXPANDS.
8. REPEAT ABOUT ONCE EACH 5 SECONDS.
    CONTINUE UNTIL BREATHING IS NORMAL.

AFCS FORM 114, SEP 74, PREVIOUS EDITIONS MAY BE USED.

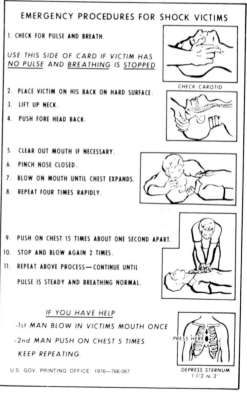

EMERGENCY PROCEDURES FOR SHOCK VICTIMS

1. CHECK FOR PULSE AND BREATH.

USE THIS SIDE OF CARD IF VICTIM HAS NO PULSE AND BREATHING IS STOPPED

CHECK CAROTID

2. PLACE VICTIM ON HIS BACK ON HARD SURFACE.
3. LIFT UP NECK.
4. PUSH FORE HEAD BACK.

5. CLEAR OUT MOUTH IF NECESSARY.
6. PINCH NOSE CLOSED.
7. BLOW ON MOUTH UNTIL CHEST EXPANDS.
8. REPEAT FOUR TIMES RAPIDLY.

9. PUSH ON CHEST 15 TIMES ABOUT ONE SECOND APART.
10. STOP AND BLOW AGAIN 2 TIMES.
11. REPEAT ABOVE PROCESS—CONTINUE UNTIL PULSE IS STEADY AND BREATHING NORMAL.

IF YOU HAVE HELP
-1st MAN BLOW IN VICTIMS MOUTH ONCE
-2nd MAN PUSH ON CHEST 5 TIMES
KEEP REPEATING.

U.S. GOV. PRINTING OFFICE: 1976—766-067

PRESS HERE

DEPRESS STERNUM 1 1/2 to 2"

The Final Responsibility

The final responsibility for determining whether or not you are physically or medically able to fly is yours alone. As the commander of your aircraft, you should know that the FAA states that "your medical certificate is legally invalid during any period of illness that prevents you from performing your flying duties properly." A good thought to keep in mind is the acronym "I'M SAFE." This little key to safety has been published by the FAA and is worth carrying as part of your checklist. The I'M SAFE personal checklist refers to *I*llness, *M*edication, *S*tress, *A*lcohol, *F*atigue, and *E*motion.

Bibliography

Armstrong, Harry G., M.D. *Aerospace Medicine*. Baltimore: Williams and Wilkins Co., 1961.

Bonfili, H.F., M.D., and Yunes, E.L., M.D. *Flight Surgeon's Check List*. San Antonio, Texas: Society of USAF Flight Surgeons, 1979.

Department of the Air Force. *Aerospace Medicine: Physiology of Flight*. Pamphlet #161-16. Washington, D.C.: Department of the Air Force, 1968.

————. *Flight Surgeon's Guide*. Pamphlet #161-18. Washington, D.C.: Department of the Air Force, 1968.

Manningham, Dan, and the Editors of *Business and Commercial Aviation* magazine. *Staying Current: A Proficiency Guide for Serious Pilots*. New York: Ziff-Davis Publishing Company, 1980.

Sharp, Wing Commander G.R. *Aviation Medicine, Physiology and Human Factors*. Edited by Air Marshal Sir Geoffrey Dhenin and Group Captain J. Ernsting. London: William Clowes & Sons Limited, 1978.

U.S. Department of Health and Human Services. *Health Information for International Travel 1978*. HEW Publication #(CDC) 78-8280. Atlanta: U.S. Department of Health, Education and Welfare, 1978.

FAR Part 67—
Medical Standards
and Certification

Appendix 1 is a reproduction of FAR Part 67—Medical Standards and Certification. This FAR is reproduced for your use in consultation, should you need official and detailed information. Under ordinary circumstances, your AME will be well acquainted with the regulations and should be able to answer questions regarding medical standards and certification.

PART 67—MEDICAL STANDARDS AND CERTIFICATION

Subpart A—General

§ 67.1 Applicability.

This subpart prescribes the medical standards for issuing medical certificates for airmen.

§ 67.11 Issue.

An applicant who meets the medical standards prescribed in this Part, based on medical examination and evaluation of his history and condition, is entitled to an appropriate medical certificate.

§ 67.13 First-class medical certificate.

a. To be eligible for a first-class medical certificate, an applicant must meet the requirements of paragraphs (b) through (f) of this section.

b. *Eye:*

1. Distant visual acuity of 20/20 or better in each eye separately, without correction; or of at least 20/100 in each eye separately corrected to 20/20 or better with corrective glasses, in which case the applicant may be qualified only on the condition that he wears those glasses while exercising the privileges of his airman certificate.
2. Near vision of at least v=1.00 at 18 inches with each eye separately, with or without corrective glasses.
3. Normal color vision.
4. Normal fields of vision.

5. No acute or chronic pathological condition of either eye or adenexae that might interfere with its proper function, might progress to that degree, or might be aggravated by flying.

6. Bifoveal fixation and vergence-phoria relationship sufficient to prevent a break in fusion under conditions that may reasonably occur in performing airman duties.

Tests for the factors named in subparagraph (6) of this paragraph are not required except for applicants found to have more than one prism diopter of hyperphoria, six prism diopters of esophoria, or six prism diopters of exophoria. If these values are exceeded, the Federal Air Surgeon may require the applicant to be examined by a qualified eye specialist to determine if there is bifoveal fixation and adequate vergencephoria relationship. However, if the applicant is otherwise qualified, he is entitled to a medical certificate pending the results of the examination.

c. *Ear, nose, throat, and equilibrium:*
1. Ability to—
   i. Hear the whispered voice at a distance of at least 20 feet with each ear separately; or
   ii. Demonstrate a hearing acuity of at least 50 percent of normal in each ear throughout the effective speech and radio range as shown by a standard audiometer.
2. No acute or chronic disease of the middle or internal ear.
3. No disease of the mastoid.
4. No unhealed (unclosed) perforation of the eardrum.
5. No disease or malformation of the nose or throat that might interfere with, or be aggravated by, flying.
6. No disturbance in equilibrium.

d. *Mental and neurologic:*
1. Mental.
   i. No established medical history or clinical diagnosis of any of the following:
      a. A personality disorder that is severe enough to have repeatedly manifested itself by overt acts.
      b. A psychosis.
      c. Alcoholism. As used in this section, "alcoholism" means a condition in which a person's intake of alcohol is great enough to damage his physical health or personal or social functioning, or when alcohol has become a prerequisite to his normal functioning.
      d. Drug dependence. As used in this section, "drug dependence" means a condition in which a person is addicted to or dependent on drugs other than alcohol, tobacco, or ordinary caffeine-containing beverages, as evidenced by habitual use or a clear sense of need for the drug.
   ii. No other personality disorder, neurosis, or mental condition that the Federal Air Surgeon finds—
      a. Makes the applicant unable to safely perform the duties or exercise the privileges of the airman certificate that he holds or for which he is applying; or
      b. May reasonably be expected,

within two years after the finding, to make him unable to perform those duties or exercise those privileges; and the findings are based on the case history and appropriate, qualified, medical judgment relating to the condition involved.

2. Neurologic.
   i. No established medical history or clinical diagnosis of either of the following:
      a. Epilepsy.
      b. A disturbance of consciousness without satisfactory medical explanation of the cause.
   ii. No other convulsive disorder, disturbance of consciousness, or neurologic condition that the Federal Air Surgeon finds—
      a. Makes the applicant unable to safely perform the duties or exercise the privileges of the airman certificate that he holds or for which he is applying; or
      b. May reasonably be expected, within two years after the finding, to make him unable to perform those duties or exercise those privileges; and the findings are based on the case history and appropriate, qualified, medical judgment relating to the condition involved.

e. *Cardiovascular:*
1. No established medical history or clinical diagnosis of—
   i. Myocardial infarction; or
   ii. Angina pectoris or other evidence of coronary heart disease that the Federal Air Surgeon finds may reasonably be expected to lead to myocardial infarction.
2. If the applicant has passed his thirty-fifth birthday but not his fortieth, he must, on the first examination after his thirty-fifth birthday, show an absence of myocardial infarction on electrocardiographic examination.
3. If the applicant has passed his fortieth birthday, he must annually show an absence of myocardial infarction on electrocardiographic examination.
4. Unless the adjusted maximum readings apply, the applicant's reclining blood pressure may not be more than the maximum reading for his age group in the following table:

AGE GROUP	MAXIMUM READINGS (RECLINING BLOOD PRESSURE IN MM)		ADJUSTED MAXIMUM READINGS (RECLINING BLOOD PRESSURE IN MM)[1]	
	SYSTOLIC	DIASTOLIC	SYSTOLIC	DIASTOLIC
20–29	140	88	—	—
30–39	145	92	155	98
40–49	155	96	165	100
50 and over	160	98	170	100

[1] For an applicant at least 30 years of age whose reclining blood pressure is more than the maximum reading for his age group and whose cardiac and kidney conditions, after complete cardiovascular examination, are found to be normal.

5. If the applicant is at least 40 years of age, he must show a degree of circulatory efficiency that is compatible with the safe operation of aircraft at high altitudes.

An electrocardiogram, made according to acceptable standards and techniques within the 90 days before an examination for a first-class certificate, is accepted at the time of the physical examination as meeting the requirements of subparagraphs (2) and (3) of this paragraph.

f. *General medical condition:*

1. No established medical history or clinical diagnosis of diabetes mellitus that requires insulin or any other hypoglycemic drug for control.

2. No other organic, functional, or structural disease, defect, or limitation that the Federal Air Surgeon finds—

   i. Makes the applicant unable to safely perform the duties or exercise the privileges of the airman certificate that he holds or for which he is applying; or

   ii. May reasonably be expected, within two years after the finding, to make him unable to perform those duties or exercise those privileges;

and the findings are based on the case history and appropriate, qualified, medical judgment relating to the condition involved.

§ 67.15 Second-class medical certificate.

a. To be eligible for a second-class medical certificate, an applicant must meet the requirements of paragraphs (b) through (f) of this section.

b. *Eye:*

1. Distant visual acuity of 20/20 or better in each eye separately, without correction; or at least 20/100 in each eye separately corrected to 20/20 or better with corrective glasses, in which case the applicant may be qualified only on the condition that he wears those glasses while exercising the privileges of his airman certificate.

2. Enough accommodation to pass a test prescribed by the Administrator based primarily on ability to read official aeronautical maps.

3. Normal fields of vision.

4. No pathology of the eye.

5. Ability to distinguish aviation signal red, aviation signal green, and white.

6. Bifoveal fixation and vergence-phoria relationship sufficient to prevent a break in fusion under conditions that may reasonably occur in performing airman duties.

Tests for the factors named in subparagraph (6) of this paragraph are not required except for applicants found to have more than one prism diopter of hyperphoria, six prism diopters of esophoria, or six prism diopters of exophoria. If these values are exceeded, the Federal Air Surgeon may require the applicant to be examined by a qualified eye specialist to determine if there is bifoveal fixation and adequate vergencephoria relationship. However, if the applicant is otherwise qualified, he is entitled to a medical certificate pending the results of the examination.

c. *Ear, nose, throat, and equilibrium:*

1. Ability to hear the whispered voice at 8 feet with each ear separately.

2. No acute or chronic disease of the middle or internal ear.

3. No disease of the mastoid.

4. No unhealed (unclosed) perforation of the eardrum.

5. No disease or malformation of the nose or throat that might interfere with, or be aggravated by, flying.

6. No disturbance in equilibrium.

d. *Mental and neurologic:*

1. Mental.

   i. No established medical history

or clinical diagnosis of any of the following:

a. A personality disorder that is severe enough to have repeatedly manifested itself by overt acts.

b. A psychosis.

c. Alcoholism. As used in this section, "alcoholism" means a condition in which a person's intake of alcohol is great enough to damage his physical health or personal or social functioning, or when alcohol has become a prerequisite to his normal functioning.

d. Drug dependence. As used in this section, "drug dependence" means a condition in which a person is addicted to or dependent on drugs other than alcohol, tobacco, or ordinary caffeine-containing beverages, as evidenced by habitual use or a clear sense of need for the drug.

ii. No other personality disorder, neurosis, or mental condition that the Federal Air Surgeon finds—

a. Makes the applicant unable to safely perform the duties or exercise the privileges of the airman certificate that he holds or for which he is applying; or

b. May reasonably be expected, within two years after the finding, to make him unable to perform those duties or exercise those privileges;

and the findings are based on the case history and appropriate, qualified, medical judgment relating to the condition involved.

2. Neurologic.

i. No established medical history or clinical diagnosis of either of the following:

a. Epilepsy.

b. A disturbance of consciousness without satisfactory medical explanation of the cause.

ii. No other convulsive disorder, disturbance of consciousness, or neurologic condition that the Federal Air Surgeon finds—

a. Makes the applicant unable to safely perform the duties or exercise the privileges of the airman certificate that he holds or for which he is applying; or

b. May reasonably be expected, within two years after the finding, to make him unable to perform those duties or exercise those privileges;

and the findings are based on the case history and appropriate, qualified, medical judgment relating to the condition involved.

e. *Cardiovascular:*

1. No established medical history or clinical diagnosis of—

i. Myocardial infarction; or

ii. Angina pectoris or other evidence of coronary heart disease that the Federal Air Surgeon finds may reasonably be expected to lead to myocardial infarction.

f. *General medical condition:*

1. No established medical history or

clinical diagnosis of diabetes mellitus that requires insulin or any other hypoglycemic drug for control.

2. No other organic, functional, or structural disease, defect, or limitation that the Federal Air Surgeon finds—

  i. Makes the applicant unable to safely perform the duties or exercise the privileges of the airman certificate that he holds or for which he is applying; or

  ii. May reasonably be expected, within 2 years after the finding to make him unable to perform those duties or exercise those privileges;

and the findings are based on the case history and appropriate, qualified, medical judgment relating to the condition involved.

§ 67.17 Third-class medical certificate.

a. To be eligible for a third-class medical certificate, an applicant must meet the requirements of paragraphs (b) through (f) of this section.

b. *Eye:*

1. Distant visual acuity of 20/50 or better in each eye separately, without correction; or if the vision in either or both eyes is poorer than 20/50 and is corrected to 20/30 or better in each eye with corrective glasses, the applicant may be qualified on the condition that he wears those glasses while exercising the privileges of his airman certificate.

2. No serious pathology of the eye.

3. Ability to distinguish aviation signal red, aviation signal green, and white.

c. *Ears, nose, throat, and equilibrium:*

1. Ability to hear the whispered voice at 3 feet.

2. No acute or chronic disease of the internal ear.

3. No disease or malformation of the nose or throat that might interfere with, or be aggravated by, flying.

4. No disturbance in equilibrium.

d. *Mental and neurologic:*

1. Mental.

  i. No established medical history or clinical diagnosis of any of the following:

    a. A personality disorder that is severe enough to have repeatedly manifested itself by overt acts.

    b. A psychosis.

    c. Alcoholism. As used in this section, "alcoholism" means a condition in which a person's intake of alcohol is great enough to damage his physical health or personal or social functioning, or when alcohol has become a prerequisite to his normal functioning.

    d. Drug dependence. As used in this section, "drug dependence" means a condition in which a person is addicted to or dependent on drugs other than alcohol, tobacco, or ordinary caffeine-containing beverages, as evidenced by habitual use or clear sense of need for the drug.

  ii. No other personality disorder, neurosis, or mental condition that the Federal Air Surgeon finds—

a. Makes the applicant unable to safely perform the duties or exercise the privileges of the airman certificate that he holds or for which he is applying; or

b. May reasonably be expected, within two years after the finding, to make him unable to perform those duties or exercise those privileges;

and the findings are based on the case history and appropriate, qualified, medical judgment relating to the condition involved.

2. Neurologic.
   i. No established medical history or clinical diagnosis of either of the following:
      a. Epilepsy.
      b. A disturbance of consciousness without satisfactory medical explanation of the cause.
   ii. No other convulsive disorder, disturbance of consciousness, or neurologic condition that the Federal Air Surgeon finds—
      a. Makes the applicant unable to safely perform the duties or exercise the privileges of the airman certificate that he holds or for which he is applying; or
      b. May reasonably be expected, within two years after the finding, to make him unable to perform those duties or exercise those privileges;
   and the findings are based on the case history and appropriate,

qualified, medical judgment relating to the condition involved.

e. *Cardiovascular:*
   1. No established medical history or clinical diagnosis of—
      i. Myocardial infarction; or
      ii. Angina pectoris or other evidence of coronary heart disease that the Federal Air Surgeon finds may reasonably be expected to lead to myocardial infarction.

f. *General medical condition:*
   1. No established medical history or clinical diagnosis of diabetes mellitus that requires insulin or any other hypoglycemic drug for control;
   2. No other organic, functional or structural disease, defect, or limitation that the Federal Air Surgeon finds—
      i. Makes the applicant unable to safely perform the duties or exercise the privileges of the airman certificate that he holds or for which he is applying; or
      ii. May reasonably be expected, within 2 years after the finding, to make him unable to perform those duties or exercise those privileges;
   and the findings are based on the case history and appropriate, qualified, medical judgment relating to the condition involved.

§ 67.19 Special issue: operational limitations.

a. A medical certificate of the appropriate class may be issued to an applicant who does not meet the medical standards of this Part, under the following procedures:

1. The Federal Air Surgeon may in his discretion find that a special medical flight or practical test, or special medical evaluation, should be conducted to determine whether the applicant can perform his duties under the airman certificate he holds, or for which he is applying, in a manner that will not endanger safety in air commerce during the period the certificate would be in force. Upon such a finding, the Federal Air Surgeon authorizes the conduct of that test or evaluation. The Federal Air Surgeon may also consider the applicant's operational experience for this purpose.

2. If the Federal Air Surgeon authorizes a procedure under subparagaph (1) of this paragraph, the applicant must show to the satisfaction of the Federal Air Surgeon, by the prescribed procedure, that he can perform those duties in the manner referred to in subparagraph (1). Upon such a showing, the Federal Air Surgeon issues to the applicant a medical certificate of the appropriate class.

b. Any operational limitation on, or limit on the duration of, a certificate issued under this section that the Federal Air Surgeon determines is needed for safety shall be specified on the airman or medical certificate held by, or issued to, the applicant.

c. An applicant who has taken a practical or flight test for a medical certificate under this section, and who has had a medical certificate issued to him under this section as a result of that test, need not take the test again during later physical examinations unless the Federal Air Surgeon determines that his physical deficiency has become enough more pronounced to require such an additional test.

d. Except for air traffic control tower operators, this section does not apply to an applicant who fails to meet the requirements of §§ 67.13(d)(1)(i), (d)(2)(i), (e)(1), or (f)(1), 67.15(d)(1)(i), (d)(2)(i), (e), or (f)(1), or 67.17(d)(1)(i), (d)(2)(i), (e), or (f)(1). A medical certificate issued to an air traffic control tower operator who does not meet the requirements of any of those sections is valid only for performing air traffic control tower operator duties.

e. The authority exercised by the Federal Air Surgeon under paragraphs (a), (b), and (c) of this section is also exercised by the Chief, Aeromedical Certification Branch, Civil Aeromedical Institute, and each Regional Flight Surgeon.

§ 67.20 Applications, certificates, logbooks, reports, and records: falsification, reproduction, or alteration.

a. No person may make or cause to be made—

1. Any fraudulent or intentionally false statement on any application for a medical certificate under this Part;

2. Any fraudulent or intentionally false entry in any logbook, record, or report that is required to be kept, made, or used, to show compliance with any requirement for any medical certificate under this Part;

3. Any reproduction, for fraudulent

purpose, of any medical certificate under this Part; or

4. Any alteration of any medical certificate under this Part.

b. The commission by any person of an act prohibited under paragraph (a) of this section is a basis for suspending or revoking any airman, ground instructor, or medical certificate or rating held by that person.

Subpart B—Certification Procedures

§ 67.21 Applicability.

This subpart prescribes the general procedures that apply to the issue of medical certificates for airmen.

§ 67.23 Medical examinations: who may give.

a. *First class.* Any aviation medical examiner who is specifically designated for the purpose may give the examination for the first class certificate. Any interested person may obtain a list of these aviation medical examiners, in any area, from the FAA Regional Director of the region in which the area is located.

b. *Second class and third class.* Any aviation medical examiner may give the examination for the second or third class certificate. Any interested person may obtain a list of aviation medical examiners, in any area, from the FAA Regional Director of the region in which the area is located.

§ 67.25 Delegation of authority.

a. The authority of the Administrator, under section 602 of the Federal Avia-

tion Act of 1958 (49 U.S.C. 1422), to issue or deny medical certificates is delegated to the Federal Air Surgeon, to the extent necessary to—

1. Examine applicants for and holders of medical certificates for compliance with applicable medical standards; and

2. Issue, renew, or deny medical certificates to applicants and holders based upon compliance or noncompliance with applicable medical standards.

Subject to limitations in this chapter, the authority delegated in subparagraphs (1) and (2) of this paragraph is also delegated to aviation medical examiners and to authorized representatives of the Federal Air Surgeon within the FAA.

b. The authority of the Administrator, under subsection 314(b) of the Federal Aviation Act of 1958 (49 U.S.C. 1355(b)), to reconsider the action of an aviation medical examiner is delegated to the Federal Air Surgeon, the Chief, Aeromedical Certification Branch, Civil Aeromedical Institute, and each Regional Flight Surgeon. Except where the applicant does not meet the standards of §§ 67.13(d)(1)(i), (d)(2)(i), (e)(1), or (f)(1), 67.15(d)(1)(i), (d)(2)(i), (e), or (f)(1), or 67.17(d)(1)(i), (d)(2)(i), (e), or (f)(1), any action taken under this paragraph other than by the Federal Air Surgeon is subject to reconsideration by the Federal Air Surgeon.

A certificate issued by an aviation medical examiner is considered to be affirmed as issued unless an FAA official named in this paragraph on his own initiative reverses that issuance within 60 days after the date of issuance. However, if within 60 days after the date of issuance that official requests the certificate holder to submit additional medical information, he may on his own initiative reverse the issuance within 60 days after he receives the requested information.

c. The authority of the Administrator, under section 609 of the Federal Aviation Act of 1958 (49 U.S.C. 1429), to reexamine any civil airman, to the extent necessary to determine an airman's qualification to continue to hold an airman medical certificate, is delegated to the Federal Air Surgeon and his authorized representatives within the FAA.

§ 67.27 Denial of medical certificate.

a. Any person who is denied a medical certificate by an aviation medical examiner may, within 30 days after the date of the denial, apply in writing and in duplicate to the Federal Air Surgeon, Attention: Chief, Aeromedical Certification Branch, Civil Aeromedical Institute, Federal Aviation Administration, P.O. Box 25082, Oklahoma City, Okla. 73125, for reconsideration of that denial. If he does not apply for reconsideration during the 30 day period after the date of the denial, he is considered to have withdrawn his application for a medical certificate.

b. The denial of a medical certificate—
   1. By an aviation medical examiner is not a denial by the Administrator under section 602 of the Federal Aviation Act of 1958 (49 U.S.C. 1422);

   2. By the Federal Air Surgeon is considered to be a denial by the Administrator under that section of the Act; and
   3. By the Chief, Aeromedical Certification Branch, Civil Aeromedical Institute, or a Regional Flight Surgeon is considered to be a denial by the Administrator under that section of the Act where the applicant does not meet the standards of §§ 67.13(d)(1)(i), (d)(2)(i), (e)(1), or (f)(1), 67.15(d)(1)(i), (d) (2)(i), (e), or (f)(1), or 67.17(d)(1)(i), (d)(2)(i), (e), or (f)(1).

Any action taken under § 67.25(b) that wholly or partly reverses the issue of a medical certificate by an aviation medical examiner is the denial of a medical certificate under this paragraph (b).

c. If the issue of a medical certificate is wholly or partly reversed upon reconsideration by the Federal Air Surgeon, the Chief, Aeromedical Certification Branch, Civil Aeromedical Institute, or a Regional Flight Surgeon, the person holding that certificate shall surrender it, upon request of the FAA.

§ 67.29 Medical certificates by senior flight surgeons of Armed Forces.

a. The FAA has designated senior flight surgeons of the Armed Forces on specified military posts, stations, and facilities, as aviation medical examiners.

b. An aviation medical examiner described in paragraph (a) of this section may give physical examinations to applicants for FAA medical certificates who are on active duty or who are, under Department of Defense medical programs, eligible for FAA medical certification as civil airmen. In addition, such an examiner may issue or deny an appropriate FAA medical certificate in accordance with the regulations of this chapter and the policies of the FAA.

c. Any interested person may obtain a list of the military posts, stations and facilities at which a senior flight surgeon has been designated as an aviation medical examiner, from the Surgeon General of the Armed Force concerned or from the Chief, Aeromedical Certification Branch, AC–130, Department of Transportation, Federal Aviation Administration, Civil Aeromedical Institute, P.O. Box 25082, Oklahoma City, Oklahoma 73125.

§ 67.31 Medical records.

Whenever the Administrator finds that additional medical information or history is necessary to determine whether an applicant for or the holder of a medical certificate meets the medical standards for it, he requests that person to furnish that information or authorize any clinic, hospital, doctor, or other person to release to the Administrator any available information or records concerning that history. If the applicant, or holder, refuses to provide the requested medical information or history or to authorize the release so requested, the Administrator may suspend, modify, or revoke any medical certificate that he holds or may, in the case of an applicant, refuse to issue a medical certificate to him.

Aviation Medical Films

The FAA makes available, at no charge, 16 millimeter sound color films for viewing by your pilot organizations. There currently are eight films available concerning aviation medicine. To order these films, make requests to Film Library, AAC–44E, Federal Aviation Administration, P.O. Box 25082, Oklahoma City, OK 73125. The films available in aviation medicine are:

- *All It Takes Is Once*
- *Charlie*
- *Disorientation*
- *Eagle-Eyed Pilot*
- *Hypoxia*
- *Medical Facts for Pilots*
- *Restraint for Survival*
- *Rx for Flight*

A description of these films is as follows:

All It Takes Is Once
Even the best of pilots can be distracted in flight by preoccupation with personal problems. Mental distraction is a serious flight hazard. How five psychological problems frequently encountered by general aviation pilots affect their performance is dramatically presented here.

Charlie
Dr. Charles Preston is a physician and should be the first to know that flying and drinking don't mix. Like a lot of us, he enjoys a drink, but doesn't adhere to the sensible "eight hours from bottle-to-throttle" rule. Charlie's judgment—and his life—are changed by alcohol, even a little of it.

Disorientation
It's important for the pilot to be aware of the fallibility of his senses and the importance of using his instruments. This aeromedical safety film alerts the pilot to inflight situations that are potentially disorienting by describing how this physiological phenomenon influences and often distorts flying judgments. The film suggests that when the physical senses are at variance with cockpit instruments, pilots should believe their instruments, not their impulses.

Eagle-Eyed Pilot
The eagle is acclaimed for its keen eyesight and superior flying ability. This film, beautifully photographed in Alaska, stresses that a pilot's "eagle" vision and flight safety go hand-in-

hand. It acquaints the general aviation pilot with the physiology of pilot vision, particularly highlighting the limitations of the eye in flight and factors that can affect and impair sight and safety while airborne.

Hypoxia

Air, air, all around; yet the pilot may be threatened and in fact debilitated by insufficient oxygen, or hypoxia. Because the body has no built-in alarm system, it is particularly important for the pilot to be aware of the danger of hypoxia and its subtle and insidious symptoms. The film shows the simple precautionary steps pilots should take to avert the threat of hypoxia.

Medical Facts for Pilots

Directed particularly to beginning pilots, this film provides a look at some of the fundamental physical, physiological, and psychological limitations in flight. It alerts pilots to such aeromedical factors as disorientation, the effects of alcohol, oxygen requirements, and pilot vision.

Restraint for Survival

Starting with dramatic highlights from the Indianapolis 500, this film demonstrates the life-saving potential of shoulder harnesses and seat belts. Documents FAA aeromedical research which simulates aircraft accidents using electronically outfitted "dummies." Suitable for showing at flight safety seminars and motor vehicle safety meetings.

Rx for Flight

Alcohol, drugs, hypoxia, disorientation, smoking, and safety equipment all lend themselves to a discussion of the basic aeromedical problems that confront general aviation pilots. This film is recommended for private pilot training classes and flight safety seminars.

PERSONAL
WEIGHT CONTROL

The chart below shows ideal weights for men and women with a variety of frame sizes and of different heights. These weights are a good approximation of where you should be. If you find that you are overweight, you suffer from one of the most common disorders in America and the one disorder which is more life-threatening than any other. Should you not comply with the weights listed in this table, you should consider a diet or over-weight program as described later in this appendix.

Below is a suggested diet-for-overweight program which will allow you to structure your foods in order to effect a weight loss. Bear in mind that the bottom line is the relationship of your calorie intake to your body use. Young people—especially those who are more active—will tend to use up more calories. A good rule of thumb is to plan to lose at least three pounds per week.

IDEAL WEIGHTS
for Men and Women—Age 25 and Over

MEN Weights in Pounds (as ordinarily dressed)

HEIGHT (WITH SHOES) FEET	INCHES	SMALL FRAME	MEDIUM FRAME	LARGE FRAME
5	2	116–125	124–133	131–142
5	3	119–128	127–136	133–144
5	4	122–132	130–140	137–149
5	5	126–136	134–144	141–153
5	6	129–139	137–147	145–157
5	7	133–143	141–151	149–162
5	8	136–147	145–156	153–166
5	9	140–151	149–160	157–170
5	10	144–155	153–164	161–175
5	11	148–159	157–168	165–180
6	0	152–164	161–173	169–185
6	1	157–169	166–178	174–190
6	2	163–175	171–184	179–196
6	3	168–180	176–189	184–202

WOMEN Weights in Pounds (as ordinarily dressed)

HEIGHT (WITH SHOES) FEET	INCHES	SMALL FRAME	MEDIUM FRAME	LARGE FRAME
5	0	105–113	112–120	119–129
5	1	107–115	114–122	121–131
5	2	110–118	117–125	124–135
5	3	113–121	120–128	127–138
5	4	116–125	124–132	131–142
5	5	119–128	127–135	133–145
5	6	123–132	130–140	138–150
5	7	126–136	134–144	142–154
5	8	129–139	137–147	145–158
5	9	133–143	141–151	149–162
5	10	136–147	145–155	152–166
5	11	139–150	148–158	155–169
6	0	141–153	151–163	160–174

(Source: Flight Surgeon's Check List)

SUGGESTED DIET FOR OVERWEIGHT PROGRAM

No substitutions are allowed on this menu. All of the asterisked items must be eaten at the meal specified. (Men may add another slice of bread at breakfast and lunch, another two ounces of meat at dinner, and two extra fruits during the day.)

Breakfast

4 oz orange or grapefruit juice, or ½ grapefruit or other high vitamin C fruit (counts as one of three daily fruits)

*1 egg or 1 oz hard cheese, or 2 oz fish, or ¼ cup cottage, pot or farmer cheese

*1 slice bread

Beverage if desired

Lunch

*4 oz fish (canned or fresh), lean meat or poultry, or ⅔ cup cottage or pot cheese, or 4 oz farmer cheese, or 2 oz hard cheese, or 2 eggs

All you want of free vegetables

*1 slice bread

Beverage if desired

Dinner

*6 oz cooked lean meat, fish or poultry

*4 oz portion any vegetable not on free list (except corn or potatoes)

All you want of free vegetables

Beverage if desired

Sometime During the Day

2 8 oz glasses powdered skim milk or buttermilk, or 1 8-oz glass skimmed evaporated milk

3 fruits

12-oz glass tomato juice (optional)

FREE FOODS

bouillon	cauliflower
low caloric carbon-	celery
ated beverage	cucumber
coffee	endive
horseradish	escarole
mustard	lettuce
salt, pepper,	mushrooms
paprika	peppers

soy sauce	pickles
tea	radishes
unflavored gelatin	rhubarb
asparagus	sauerkraut
bean sprouts	spinach
beans, french style	squash, summer
broccoli	watercress
cabbage	

FORBIDDEN FOODS

alcoholic beverages	gravy
avocado	honey
bacon or fat back	ice cream or ices
beer	jam, jelly
biscuits	mayonnaise
butter	muffins
cake	nuts
candy	oils
carbonated bever-	olives
ages (except	pancakes
noncaloric)	peanut butter
catsup	pie
cereals	popcorn
chocolate	pretzels
coconut	pudding
cookies	rice
corn	rolls, special
crackers	breads
cream (sweet or	salad dressing
sour)	sardines
cream cheese	smoked fish or
doughnuts	meat
fried foods	spaghetti
fruit-flavored	sugar, syrup
gelatin	waffles

(Source—Flight Surgeon's Check List)

Below is a calorie counter of common foods. Calories can be reduced by substituting similar foods noted in the second column. This results in a significant calorie saving, as noted in the third column.

CALORIE COUNTER

FOR THIS	CALORIES	SUBSTITUTE THIS	CALORIES	CALORIES SAVED
MEATS				
Loin Roast, 3½ oz.	340	Pot Roast (Round), 3½ oz.	200	140
Rump Roast, 3½ oz.	340	Rib Roast, 3½ oz.	260	80
Swiss Steak, 3½ oz.	300	Liver (fried), 3½ oz.	210	90
Hamburger (av. fat, brld.), 3 oz.	245	Lean, broiled, 3 oz.	185	60
Porterhouse Steak, 3½ oz.	290	Club Steak, 3½ oz.	190	100
Rib Lamb Chop (medium), 3 oz.	300	Lamb Leg Roast, 3 oz.	235	65
Pork Chop (medium), 3 oz.	340	Veal Chop (medium), 3 oz.	185	155
Pork Roast, 3 oz.	310	Veal Roast, 3 oz.	230	80
Pork Sausage, 3 oz.	405	Ham (boiled, lean), 3 oz.	200	205
POTATOES				
Potatoes (fried), 1 cup	480	Baked, 2½" diameter	100	380
Potatoes (mashed), 1 cup	240	Boiled, 2½" diameter	100	140
SALADS				
Chef Salad/Regular oil, 1 T.	160	With Dietetic Dressing, 1 T.	40	120
Chef Salad/Mayonnaise, 1 T.	125	With Dietetic Dressing, 1 T.	40	85
Chef Salad/French, Russian, Roquefort, 1 T.	105	With Dietetic Dressing, 1 T.	40	65
SANDWICHES				
Club Sandwich	375	Open Bacon & Tomato	200	175
Peanut Butter and Jelly	275	Egg Salad	165	110
Turkey with Gravy	300	Open Hamburger (lean), 2 oz.	200	100
SNACKS				
Fudge, 1 oz.	115	Vanilla Wafers, dietetic, 2	50	65
Peanuts (salted), 1 oz.	190	Apple, 1	70	120
Peanuts (roasted), 1 cup	800	Grapes, 1 cup	65	735
Potato Chips, 10 med. chips	115	Pretzels, 10 small sticks	35	80
Chocolate, 1 oz. bar	145	Marshmallows, 3	60	85
SOUPS				
Creamed soup, 1 cup	135	Chicken Noodle soup, 1 cup	65	70
Bean soup, 1 cup	170	Beef Noodle soup, 1 cup	70	100
Minestrone soup, 1 cup	105	Beef Bouillon, 1 cup	30	75
VEGETABLES				
Baked Beans, 1 cup	320	Green Beans, 1 cup	30	290
Lima Beans, 1 cup	180	Asparagus, 1 cup	35	145

FOR THIS	CALORIES	SUBSTITUTE THIS	CALORIES	CALORIES SAVED
Corn (canned), 1 cup	170	Cauliflower, 1 cup	25	145
Peas (canned), 1 cup	165	Peas (fresh), 1 cup	115	50
Winter Squash, 1 cup	130	Summer Squash, 1 cup	30	100
Succotash, 1 cup	260	Spinach, 1 cup	40	220
BEVERAGES				
Milk (whole), 8 oz.	160	Buttermilk, Skim, 8 oz.	90	70
Prune Juice, 8 oz.	200	Tomato Juice, 8 oz.	45	155
Soft Drinks, 8 oz.	105	Diet Soft Drinks, 8 oz.	1	104
Coffee (cream & 2 tsp. sugar)	95	Coffee (Blk/artificial sugar)	0	95
Cocoa (all milk), 8 oz.	235	Cocoa (milk & water), 8 oz.	140	95
Chocolate Malted, 8 oz.	450	Lemonade (sweetened), 8 oz.	100	350
Beer (1 bottle), 12 oz.	185	Liquor/soda or water, 8 oz.	150	35
BREAKFAST FOODS				
Rice Flakes, 1 cup	105	Puffed Rice, 1 cup	55	50
Eggs (scrambled), 2	220	Boiled or poached, 2	160	60
BUTTER AND CHEESE				
Butter on toast	170	Apple Butter on toast	90	80
Cheese (Blue, Cheddar, Cream, Swiss), 1 oz.	105	Cheese (Cottage, uncreamed), 1 oz.	25	80
DESSERTS				
Angel Food Cake, 2" piece	110	Cantaloupe Melon, ½ melon	60	50
Cheese Cake, 2" piece	200	Watermelon, ½" slice	60	140
Chocolate Cake, iced, 2" pc.	445	Sponge Cake, 2" piece	120	325
Fruit Cake, 2" piece	115	Grapes, 1 cup	65	50
Pound Cake, 1 oz. piece	140	Plums, 2	50	90
Iced Cupcake, 1	185	Plain Cupcake, 1	145	40
Cookies, assorted, 3" dia., 1	120	Vanilla Wafer (dietetic), 1	25	95
Ice Cream, 4 oz.	150	Yogurt (flavored), 4 oz.	60	90
Pie, Apple, 1/7 pc. of 9" pie	345	Tangerine (fresh), 1	40	305
Pie, Blueberry, 1 piece	290	Blueberries (frozen, unsweetened), ½ cup	45	245
Pie, Cherry, 1 piece	355	Cherries (fresh, whole), ½ cup	40	315
Pie, Custard, 1 piece	280	Banana, 1	85	195
Pie, Lemon Meringue, 1 piece	305	Lemon flav. gelatin, ½ c.	70	235
Pie, Peach, 1 piece	280	Peach (fresh), 1	35	245
Pie, Rhubarb, 1 piece	265	Grapefruit, ½	55	210
Pudding (flavored), ½ cup	140	Dietetic, non-fat milk, ½ c.	60	80

FOR THIS	CALORIES	SUBSTITUTE THIS	CALORIES	CALORIES SAVED
FISH AND FOWL				
Tuna (canned), 3 oz.	170	Crabmeat (canned), 3 oz.	85	85
Oysters (fried), 6	250	On shell with sauce, 6	100	150
Ocean Perch (fried), 4 oz.	260	Bass, 4 oz.	105	155
Fish Sticks, 5 sticks or 4 oz.	200	Brook Trout, 4 oz.	130	70
Lobster, (2 T. butter), 4 oz.	300	Lobster, 4 oz./lemon	95	205
Duck (roasted), 4 oz.	200	Chicken (roasted), 4 oz.	140	60

(Source—Flight Surgeon's Check List)

The calorie value of common snack foods is shown in the chart below. The real danger in snack foods is that most provide an inordinate number of calories, which we frequently ingest above and beyond our regular meals, but little nutri-tion. Some items, such as a malted milk with 450 calories, could equal a total meal—if the meal were properly structured. The trick is to avoid snacks and eat three balanced regular meals each day.

CALORIC VALUES FOR COMMON SNACK FOODS

BEVERAGES	AMOUNT OR AVERAGE SERVING	CALORIE COUNT	PROTEIN GRAMS
Carbonated drinks, soda, root beer, etc............................	6 oz. glass	80	0
Club soda......................	8 oz. glass	5	0
Chocolate malted milk	10 oz. glass (1¾ cups)	450	11.5
Ginger ale	6 oz. glass	60	0
Tea or coffee, straight	1 cup	0	0
Tea or coffee, with 2 tablespoonfuls cream and 2 teaspoonfuls sugar .	1 cup	90	0.8
ALCOHOLIC DRINKS			
1 Ale	8 oz. glass	130	0.9
1 Beer	8 oz. glass	110	0.9
1 Highball......................	8 oz. glass	140	0
1 Manhattan....................	Average	175	0
1 Martini	Average	160	0
1 Old Fashioned	Average	150	0
1 Sherry	2 oz. glass	60	0.2
Scotch, bourbon, rye	1 oz. jigger	80	0

FRUITS	AMOUNT OR AVERAGE SERVING	CALORIE COUNT	PROTEIN GRAMS
Apple	1 3-inch	90	.5
Banana	1 6-inch	100	1.2
Grapes	30 medium	75	1.0
Orange	1 2¾-inch	80	1.4
Pear..........................	1	100	1.0

CANDIES			
Chocolate bars			
Plain	1 bar (1¼ oz.)	190	2.0
With nuts	1 bar	275	5.0
Chocolate covered bar	1 bar	250	5.0
Chocolate cream, bonbon, fudge ..	1 piece 1" square	90	0.6
Caramels			
Plain	1 piece ¾" cubes	35	0.5
Chocolate nut caramels	1 piece	60	0.8

DESSERTS			
Pie			
Fruit........................	1/6 pie 1 average serving	560	5.5
Custard......................	1/6 pie 1 average serving	360	8.5
Lemon meringue	1/6 pie 1 average serving	470	6.0
Pumpkin pie with whipped cream	1/6 pie 1 average serving	460	8.3
Cake			
Iced layer—2 layers white cake ..	1 average serving	345	5.2
Fruit—thin slice ¼".............	1 average serving	125	1.5

SALTED NUTS			
Almonds......................	10	130	4.0
Cashews......................	10	60	2.0
Peanuts	10	60	2.7
Pecans	10 halves	150	2.0

"JUST A LITTLE SANDWICH"			
Hamburger on bun..............	3" patty	500	22.5
Peanut butter	2 tablespoonfuls P.B.	370	14.0
Cheese	1½ oz. cheese	400	14.6
Ham..........................	1½ oz. ham	350	13.0

MIDNIGHT SNACKS FOR ICE-BOX RAIDERS			
Cold potato	½ medium	65	1.5
Chicken leg	1 average	88	15.0
Milk	7 oz. glass	140	7.0
Mouthful of roast	½" × 2" × 3"	130	11.0
Piece of cheese.................	¼" × 2" × 3"	120	7.2
Left-over beans.................	½ cup	105	6.6

	AMOUNT OR AVERAGE SERVING	CALORIE COUNT	PROTEIN GRAMS
Brownie	¾″ × 1¾″ × 2¼″	300	3.9
Cream-puff	4″ diameter	450	5.7

SWEETS

Ice cream			
Plain vanilla	1/6 qt. serving	200	4.0
Chocolate and other flavors	1/6 qt., ¾ cup	230	4.5
Milk sherbet	1/6 qt., ¾ cup	250	4.0
Sundaes, small chocolate nut with			
whipped cream	Average	400	10.0
Ice cream sodas, chocolate	10 oz. glass	270	3.5

(Source—Flight Surgeon's Check List)

Alcohol

The clinical states related to a variety of alcohol levels as determined by blood analysis and/or urine analysis are summarized in the chart below. Bear in mind that the overall state and clinical state portrayed in this graph are at ground level. The effects of alcohol are poten- tiated by the hypoxia of flying at altitude, effects which are even more noticeable at night. Remember that the rule of eight hours from bottle to throttle is a mini- mum FAA requirement. A better rule is twenty-four hours.

CLINICAL STATES RELATED TO ALCOHOL LEVELS

BLOOD	URINE	OVERALL STATE	CLINICAL STATE
0.01–0.05 (10–50 mg%)	0.01–0.07	Apparently normal	No apparent influence, behavior nearly normal by ordinary ob- servation. Slight changes de- tectable by special tests.
0.03–0.12 (30–120 mg%)	0.04–0.16	Likable	Mild euphoria, sociability, talka- tiveness; increased self-confi- dence; decreased inhibitions; diminution of attention, judg- ment, and control. Loss of efficiency in finer performance tests.
0.90–0.25 (90–250 mg%)	0.12–0.34	Compromised function	Emotional instability; decreased inhibitions; loss of critical judg- ment, impairment of memory and comprehension, decreased sensory response; increased reaction time; some muscular incoordination.

BLOOD	URINE	OVERALL STATE	CLINICAL STATE
0.18–0.30 (180–300 mg%)	0.24–0.41	Obviously impaired	Disorientation, mental confusion; dizziness; exaggerated emotional states (fear, anger, grief); disturbance of sensation (diplopia) and of perception of color, form, motion, dimensions; decreased pain sense; impaired balance; muscular incoordination; staggering gait, slurred speech.
0.27–0.40 (270–400 mg%)	0.37–0.54	Helpless	Apathy; general inertia, approaching paralysis; greatly decreased response to stimuli; marked muscular incoordination, inability to stand or walk; vomiting; incontinence of urine and feces; impaired consciousness, sleep or stupor.
0.35–0.50 (350–500 mg%)	0.47–0.67	Obtunded	Complete unconsciousness, coma, anesthesia; depressed or abolished reflexes; subnormal temperature; incontinence of urine and feces; embarrassment of circulatory and respiration. Possible death.
0.45 + (450 mg% +)	0.60 +	Lethal	Death from respiratory paralysis.

(Source—Flight Surgeon's Check List)

Use the chart below to determine the approximate percentage of alcohol in the blood in relation to body weight.

The actual blood alcohol is altered by rate of absorption which depends on many variables, such as type of drink, previous food, etc.

The average rate of decrease of blood alcohol (primarily by metabolism) is .015% per hour. Therefore, .15% would require approximately ten hours to reach zero.

Depending on the extent of after effects (hangover), one cannot state that a negligible blood alcohol is necessarily commensurate with best performance capability.

(Source—FAA)

BLOOD-ALCO CHART

	DRINKS	1	2	3	4	5	6	7	8	9	10	11	12
BODY WEIGHT	100 lb.	.038	.075	.113	.150	.188	.225	.263	.300	.338	.375	.413	.450
	120 lb.	.031	.063	.094	.125	.156	.188	.219	.250	.281	.313	.344	.375
	140 lb.	.027	.054	.080	.107	.134	.161	.188	.214	.241	.268	.295	.321
	160 lb.	.023	.047	.070	.094	.117	.141	.164	.188	.211	.234	.258	.281
	180 lb.	.021	.042	.063	.083	.104	.125	.146	.167	.188	.208	.229	.250
	200 lb.	.019	.038	.056	.075	.094	.113	.131	.150	.169	.188	.206	.225
	220 lb.	.017	.034	.051	.068	.085	.102	.119	.136	.153	.170	.188	.205
	240 lb.	.016	.031	.047	.063	.078	.094	.109	.125	.141	.156	.172	.188

ICAO Rest Formula

Appendix 5 is the ICAO formula for determining rest when traveling beyond your local time zone. See the discussion of fatigue in Chapter III to learn how important appropriate rest is to the pilot.

The *ICAO formula* is as follows:

$$\text{Rest period (in tenths of days)} = \frac{\text{Travel time (hours)}}{2} + \text{Time zones excess of 4}$$

$$+ \text{Departure time coefficient (local time)} + \text{Arrival time coefficient (local time)}$$

The departure and arrival time coefficients are given in the following table.

Period	Departure time coefficient	Arrival time coefficient
0800–1159 hours	0	4
1200–1759 hours	1	2
1800–2159 hours	3	0
2200–0059 hours	4	1
0100–0800 hours	3	3

The increased weight given the later hours for departures helps compensate for the effects of loss of sleep. Also, the high arrival-time coefficient for the period 0800 to 1159 hours helps compensate for the disruptions experienced during early morning flights plus the effect of arriving at the beginning of a workday without sufficient rephasing of the circadian rhythms. The amount of phase difference is accounted for in the formula by the term "time zones in excess of 4."

In applying the formula, the following rules are observed by ICAO:

(1) The value obtained for rest period, in tenths of days, is to be rounded to the nearest higher half day. However, rest stops that add up to less than a day before rounding will not be scheduled unless the journey involves an overnight flight on mission travel.

(2) "Travel time, in hours" means the number of hours of elapsed time required for the journey rounded off to the nearest hour.

(3) "Time zones" are computed in increments of 15 degrees of longitude from Greenwich.

(4) "Departure time" and "arrival time" are local times.

Carbon Monoxide Levels

Dangerous concentrations of carbon monoxide can be fatal in less than one hour. A headache and general nausea are dangerous symptoms.

DANGEROUS CONCENTRATIONS OF CARBON MONOXIDE

CONCENTRATION, PERCENT	EFFECT
0.01, or 1 part in 10,000	No symptoms for 2 hours
0.04, or 4 parts in 10,000	No symptoms for 1 hour
0.06 to 0.07, or 6 to 7 parts in 10,000	Headache and unpleasant symptoms in 1 hour
0.10 to 0.12, or 10 to 12 parts in 10,000	Dangerous for 1 hour
0.35 or 35 parts in 10,000	Fatal in less than 1 hour

(AFP 161-16 Appendix IX)

SENSORY ILLUSIONS

Appendix 7 is a detailed report of sensory illusions by the Flight Safety Foundation. This is included to show you not only how complicated analysis of sensory illu- sions can be, but how valuable an under- standing of sensory illusions is to the pilot. (Reprinted by permission of the Flight Safety Foundation.)

SENSORY ILLUSIONS

The following paper* won for its author, Prosper Cocquyt, the 1952 Flight Safety Foundation Award. At the time, Capt. Cocquyt was Chief Pilot, Sabena Belgian World Airlines.

ENORMOUS progress has been made in the field of aviation safety. The results are particularly evident in the services of scheduled airlines. This has been accomplished through the amazing developments of science and industry, by the considerable but little known efforts of the ICAO and IATA in the field of commercial aviation and, last but not least, as a product of tne experience of all those engaged in operating aircraft.

Despite this progress, accidents due to navigation and piloting errors are still occurring. After an accident the board of inquiry is often confronted with a difficult task and is at times unable to ascertain the actual causes; in such cases the conclusion is usually reached that the accident is due to an error of judgment on the part of the pilot, and even when the pilot survives, he is, in most cases, unable to offer a valid explanation.

Fig. 1.

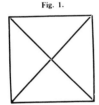

More than 30 years of personal experience—and study started in 1931—led me to the conclusion that the causes of a certain category of flight accidents ought to be sought in a phenomenon still extremely vague for most people concerned with aviation: that is, sensory illusions, and in particular optical illusions. There are a number of psychological works treating the description of sensations and perceptions. I am convinced that a thorough examination of these questions in relation to the piloting of aircraft could reveal the explanation of many flight accidents.

Some Psychological Principles

Life is full of illusions; in the majority of cases, human conceptions are purely imaginary. From birth, man, influenced by heredity, faces the outside world through the five senses: feeling, seeing, hearing, tasting and smelling. Each time a man is subjected to a sensory stimulus, an impression is made on him which gradually fades away. All these impressions shape the man and, combined with his hereditary character, form the base of human individuality.

Each new stimulus may set up a vision and give rise to a reaction; however, the resulting action will not necessarily be in direct relation to that quality of the stimulus, but may also be influenced by the state of mind of the affected individual. Effect of sensorial stimuli is norm 'ly predominant; however, in many cases, it is the intelligence which will have a predominant bearing on the effects of the visual stimuli.

• Reprinted from Shell Aviation News #178, April, 1953

Figure 1 gives a typical example; this, of course, is merely a few ink lines on a piece of paper. Visual stimuli are always identical; however, according to the state of his mind, the observer can imagine such different objects as a square with two diagonals, a group of four triangles, a pyramid with square base, a pyramidal well with square top, etc., etc. Each of these figures may be imagined with different sizes but only one figure can be seen at a time.

Observation of stars is another obvious example. To the uninformed observer, the stars appear as points of light scattered over a celestial dome. The astronomer on the other hand, sees these same points of light arranged in different planes, and can calculate their position in space, their size and special characteristics.

Another example: three lights emitting the same quantity of light energy are seen simultaneously by the pilot in a normal flight from the same angle of separation. Provided that the pilot's visual organs are perfect, these three lights ought to be seen on a circle passing a vertical plan, the radius of which

equals $1 = \dfrac{W}{4\pi}$ when 1 = intensity of light and W =

quantity of light energy. Now a threshold differential of intensity of visual stimuli is imperative for evoking a perception. As a result, in certain circumstances, particularly where there is no previous knowledge of their position, these three lights can be seen on all planes which cut the visual rays (fig. 2).

There is an infinity of illusions. Some are quite impressively and perfectly produced in music-hall shows and conjuring exhibitions.

Some Aspects of Pilots' Psychology

The pilot locates himself in space by observing landmarks outside the aircraft or by observation of applicable instruments. Proper reading of these instruments will give the pilot a correct estimation of the aircraft's position whereas observation of reference points may, under certain circumstances, be quite inadequate.

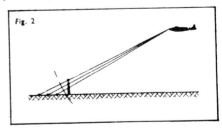

Fig. 2

Here are some examples showing what can happen if the pilot neglects to consult his instruments. Under conditions of poor visibility over an area without landmarks (sea, desert, even ground—more particularly when covered with snow, forest, etc.), the pilot is unable to determine the position of the aircraft with relation to any of the three axes of freedom (fig. 3.).

FIG. 3. AIRCRAFT'S AXIS OF FREEDOM

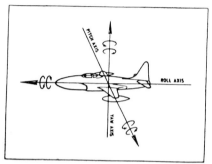

In the case of a flight over an unknown area, it is impossible to determine the position of the aircraft with relation to the yaw axis, whereas the position with respect to the rolling and pitching axes will be readily observed. At night, observation of a remote light provides an accurate sensation of its direction (yaw axis) whereas awareness of the horizontal attitude (rolling and pitching axis) and of height can be non-existent.

In the case of landing on a level surface of water, many accidents have been caused by misjudgment of height; the visual stimuli given by the observation of such a surface does not provide the pilot with adequate information for correct estimation of his relative height. Accidents occurring before reaching an airport which does not possess the appropriate landmarks in the approach sector, belong also to this category. From the above, we may infer that the nature of the visual stimuli must be such that the resulting sensation shall provide the pilot with instantaneous knowledge of his true position.

In the foregoing examples, it is assumed that the pilot is flying at a constant speed and is subject only to the force of gravity. However, in the course of certain flights, he may be subject to accelerations modifying his sensory perception of gravity force. The combined effect of the forces—i.e. gravity and acceleration—could deprive the pilot of any exact knowledge of his position in space and lead him to make errors as great as 180° in both directions, with relation to the three axes of freedom of the aircraft. It will be noted that man has no sense which allows him to discriminate between the relative effects of these two forces.

An error of 180° with respect to the yaw axis will lead the pilot in a direction exactly opposite that which he imagines. I have myself seen several cases

in which a pilot was completely out of direction. An error of 180° with relation to the rolling or pitching axis will result in inverted flight when the pilot believes his attitude to be normal. Indeed, a roll (rolling axis) or a loop (pitching axis) may eventually develop an acceleration of two g when upside down; the resulting force acting on the pilot's body is thus equal to 1 g and induces the same cenesthetic sensation as a normal horizontal flight. Numbers of errors of this nature were made in the early days of aviation when pilots flew in cloud or in other zero visibility conditions without blind flying instruments.

Nowadays, this type of error still occurs frequently, and is generally due to malfunctioning of flight instruments or to their lack of response to certain abnormal manoeuvres of the aircraft. When flying blind, the pilot is always more or less conscious of his position in respect to the ground. Without the help of his flight instruments, he may have a certain cenesthetic sensation of his position but is unable to determine it accurately. On emerging from cloud under such conditions, the visual stimuli of the ground will normally give the pilot definite indications of his true position. No readjustment is required if the initial imaginary position corresponds to the true position.

On the other hand, if the position as originally envisaged is false, a conflict arises between the initial sensation and the new one set up by the visual stimuli. If the visual stimuli are of such a nature that they eradicate the false impression, the illusion will disappear instantly, but if the stimuli are not suffi-

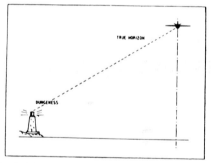

FIG. 4A (left) NORMAL FLIGHT PASSING THE LIGHTHOUSE OF DUNGENESS AND LOOKING LEFT

FIG. 4B (below) FLIGHT ALONG THE COAST AT AN ESTIMATED HEIGHT OF 300 FT.—ILLUSION OF 20° TO THE RIGHT

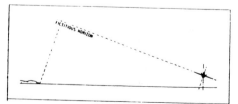

FIG. 5. 10° ILLUSION TO THE LEFT OF THE ROLL AXIS

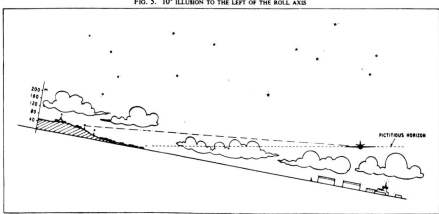

cient to establish the true position, the illusion may persist.

Here is an illusion which frequently occurs: a pilot has the sensation of flying horizontally, while, in fact, his aircraft is banked. Looking at the ground he sees the houses, the trees and other objects in a position which does not match his imagined horizon. Immediately the visual stimuli of the houses, trees and so on, whose position he knows, induce the sensation of his true position, and the false impression he previously had is instantly eliminated. The duration of the conflict between these two sensations is always extremely short.

Personal Experiences

More than twenty years ago, I realized that optical illusions might be responsible for a number of aviation accidents. On 11th September, 1930, an accident occurred to an aircraft of our Company. A tri-motored Fokker VII operating a night mail service with a pilot and flight engineer on board, turned back several minutes after take-off from Croydon, probably because of bad visibility; it crashed on the starboard wing near the airfield and caught fire.

A few months later, on 9th January, 1931, a second Fokker bound for Croydon crashed at Melle, on the right of the Ghent - Brussels road, after radioing that the aircraft was returning due to bad visibility. Conditions of the accident were similar but the aircraft did not catch fire. What struck me most was the fact that the flight engineer was found dead with both hands in the pockets of his jacket. This led to the conclusion that the crew had no advance warning and

that the accident took place without any reaction on the part of the crew.

This called to mind an incident during a night flight I once made with a pilot I was training on the Croydon-Brussels route. When passing Dungeness, I made a turn to the left around the lighthouse to fly towards Folkestone. I was flying below the clouds at an approximate altitude of 150 metres in light rain and a visibility of 1 to 2 kilometres. After this turn, I met certain difficulties in following the coastline as

FIG. 6. NORMAL FLIGHT LOOKING AT THE LIGHTHOUSE AT AN ANGLE OF 6° BELOW THE HORIZON

TRUE HORIZON

(A)

5' ILLUSION ON THE PITCHING AXIS

FICTITIOUS HORIZON

(B)

my aircraft developed a tendency to turn to the right, but I did not attach any importance to this at the time. I descended somewhat to improve my observation when the co-pilot suddenly pulled the stick, shouting that I was flying very low; he could see the reflection of the green navigation light on the sea. I estimated my altitude to be 100 metres approximately, and told him he was mistaken as I had a definite view of the coastline.

In comparing this incident with the two accidents described above, I was convinced that I must have had my aircraft banked to the right and that the co-pilot had made a correct estimation of the height in judging from the reflection of the green light in the water. My estimation of the distance to the coast was correct, but my estimation of the height above the water was completely wrong, as I had indeed the sensation of flying the aircraft in a normal attitude although it was undoubtedly banked to the right. This is the typical optical illusion with respect to the rolling axis (fig. 4))

Another case of optical illusion about the rolling axis was experienced by another crew which, on arriving at Croydon at night in good visibility above 3 to 5/10 low stratus cloud, mistook the lights of Purley for stars (fig. 5).

At about the same period, a similar accident occurred to one of our crews in course of a night flight. After leaving the British coast and flying in good visibility, towards the lighthouse of Cape Gris-Nez, the pilot reduced the engine power setting to keep below clouds. The aircraft gradually lost altitude until the trailing antenna struck the water. The crew did not realize that the angle of incidence was greater than before throttling back and therefore viewed the lighthouse below its fictitious horizon. The light gave the pilots a wrong sensation of their height, whereas the shock felt when the antenna struck the water warned them of their true position (fig. 6.)

About the same period, I studied approximately ten other night flying accidents. They had one point in common, crashing on the starboard wing after completion of a 180° left turn. Unfortunately, at that time I was unable to find a convincing explanation and my first report in connexion with this problem did not throw any new light on the matter. Since such accidents occurred repeatedly, I was convinced that many of them could have been caused by optical illusions, but I was still unable to prove it. In 1950 I prepared a second report, following a series of commercial aviation accidents. This paper attracted the attention of many aeronautical authorities, particularly after it was translated and published by the "Flight Safety Foundation" in New York.

Later the study of several recent accidents led me in January 1952 to a satisfactory mathematical explanation of the effects of illusions arising in relation to the rolling and pitching axes.

Optical illusions are always created in the course of manoeuvres when the pilot does not follow the sequence of movements of his aircraft; under such conditions, the imagined position differs from the true position. In the foregoing I have already explained how a pilot can make errors as great as 180° in both directions with respect to the three axes of freedom, when he is deprived of the knowledge of his actual position in the space. In controlling his aircraft when unwarned of his true position with relation to the three axes of freedom, the pilot will have wrong reactions which are the potential cause of accidents resulting from illusions. Nevertheless, incorrect estimation of the relative height is chiefly due to illusions about the rolling and pitching axes and is the cause of most commercial aviation accidents.

To give rise to optical illusions, the observed reference points should be presented by objects without relief and located in surroundings without relief. However, flush landmarks, when grouped to create peculiar geometrical figures, may allow proper determination of the horizontal plane.

In observing landmarks the pilot determines his relative height by estimation of the distance D to the landmarks, and the angle a between the direction of observation of the landmarks and his horizon. Angle a is normally positive as the landmarks are usually observed below his horizon; it will, however, be negative if the observed landmarks are located above his horizon. Theoretically angle a may take any value between 0 and ±180°. The angle a is always included between the direction of the observed landmarks and the pilot's true horizon. If the estimation of both the distance D and the angle a is correct, the value of the true height H may be expressed by

$$H = D \sin a$$

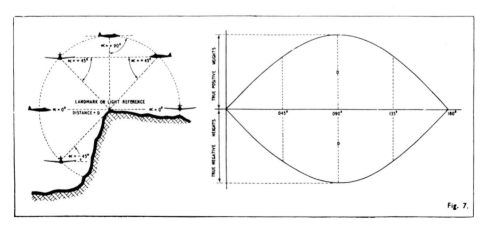

Fig. 7.

The true height is proportional to the distance from landmark D and to the sine of the angle a; for a given distance its variation is thus given by a sinusoid (fig. 7).

When the imagined position is not a reflection of the true position, the landmark is observed at an angle $(a + \theta)$, θ being the angle included between the true and the imagined horizon. This angle may also vary between 0 and ±180°.

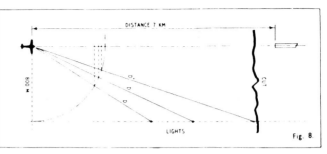

Then angle θ creates an imaginary height, which is the distance to the imaginary horizontal plane (perpendicular to the imaginary plane). The planes of the imaginary ground necessarily intersect the plane of the actual ground at the observed landmark. A row or a group of landmarks parallel to the direction of the aircraft would result in the same effect as a single landmark.

We know that the product of the sine by the cosecant of an angle is equal to the radius of the trigonometric circumference; in this case, the radius represents the distance to the landmark. Intersection of the true with the imaginary plane divides the horizon in two equal parts; it may be created in any direction; however, as already stated above, errors due to optical illusions are most likely to occur with relation to the rolling and pitching axes. Effect of illusion is maximum when observation is made perpendicular to, and minimum (zero) when it is made parallel to the intersection of the two planes (fig. 8).

Figure 9 represents the errors in height estimations resulting from optical illusions about the rolling and pitching axes with respect to a landmark or a row of landmarks; this figure clearly shows the effects of these illusions. Imaginary heights H' are proportional to distance D of landmark (as the true height) and to sine of angle $(a + \theta)$.

$$H' = D \sin (a + \theta)$$

Imaginary heights are positive or negative with respect to the true height of the aircraft, positive heights will be found for a positive angle of 180° — $2a$ (fig. 10). The ratio of imaginary height H' to the true height may be written:

$$\frac{H'}{H} = \frac{D \sin (a + \theta)}{D \sin a}$$

This expression will take determined value for a values other than 0° and 180°, thus:

$$H' = \frac{H \sin (a + \theta)}{\sin a}$$

This shows that usually the maximum effect of positive imaginary height is met when the true height

FIG. 9. ILLUSIONS OF 5° AND 10° FOR TRUE HEIGHTS OF 0-150 M. (500 FT.) AND 300 M. (1,000 FT.)

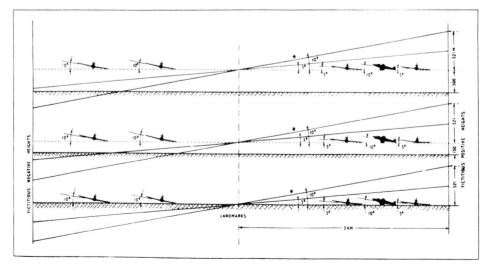

is equal to zero. In this case the positive imaginary height H' = D sin θ (positive). However, for negative true heights, maximum effect will be obtained for a = —90°. Effect of positive imaginary heights decreases proportionally to sine of angle a (positive), this height has already decreased 50% at 30° (Fig. 11) and become zero at 90°.

When imaginary heights are positive, the pilot has the sensation of flying higher than his true height. Imaginary ground is above the actual ground beyond the landmarks. Thus, in case of night flight the pilot may see stars below his imaginary ground and mistake them for ground lights. Under these conditions he may also see the runway sloped down. Serious hazard exists if an optical illusion resulting in positive imaginary height arises and persists in course of the landing procedure; for the pilot keeps on with his let down until he reaches the ground and at this point still has the sensation of flying at a height equal to H' = D sin θ. The value of this imaginary height may reach impressive figures even for relatively small angle differences. Thus, for a landmark observed from a distance of 1 km. with an illusion angle of 10°, the imaginary height will be 174 metres.

When imaginary heights are negative, the pilot has the sensation of flying lower than he actually is; under these conditions, the imaginary ground is below the actual ground beyond the landmarks and the pilot may see, at night, the ground lights above his imaginary ground and mistake them for stars. He may also see the runway sloped up.

A particular illusion will arise when the pilot believes he is flying above a row of landmarks. True height is then equal to imaginary height H' multiplied by sine of angle of illusion θ, thus distance D will be equal to H' cos θ. (fig. 12).

When a pilot is subject to an optical illusion in relation with the axis of roll and he imagines himself flying in a horizontal position, although he is flying in a rolled position, the following situation may occur:

(1) Flying just over a row of lights: *(a) with an angle of roll to the right:* In this condition the projection of his vertical plane on the ground (depending on the angle of roll and the height of his aircraft) is on the left side of the row of lights. The pilot's aim is to line up with the row of lights because this is the easiest way to follow a row of lights. By attempting to line up, the pilot will steer his aircraft still further to the right and increase the hazardous condition already existing. *(b) With an angle of roll to the left* the same conditions as in (a) occur with "right" for "left" and vice versa.

(2) Flying on the right side of the row of lights with a right angle of roll: In this condition the pilot cannot determine the part "distance to the right side of the row of lights" and the part "projection of his vertical plane." Three conditions may occur: *(a) The projection of his vertical plane is to the left side of the row of lights:* By attempting to line up, the pilot will steer further to the right and increase the hazardous condition already existing; *(b)   The projection of his vertical plane is upon the row of lights:* The pilot will not react in this condition but his aircraft will have a tendency to swing to the right. With certain aircraft the pilot may follow the row of lights with the angle of roll by holding the direction with the rudder, but normally the aircraft will swing to the right and the pilot will react by steering to the left. By doing this he will decrease the hazardous condition already existing; *(c) The projection of his vertical plane is to the right side of the row of lights:* By attempting to line up, the pilot will steer to the left and decrease the existing hazardous condition.

(3) Flying to left side of row of lights with a left angle of roll: the same conditions as in (2), (a), (b), (c) may occur with "left" for "right" and vice versa.

Apparently optical illusion about the yaw axis could not take place as landmarks cannot possibly be seen in more than one direction. Nevertheless many accidents resulting from sensory illusions with relation to aircraft path have occurred. In the course of level flight, the aircraft path is determined by movements in relation to the yaw axis. A number of

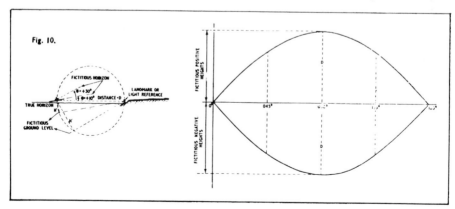

Fig. 10.

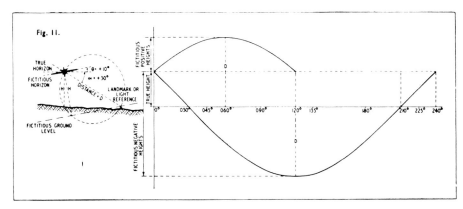

stimuli of various kinds give rise to such illusions. The stimuli do not appear to seriously affect the sensations of position; the pilot's intelligence has an overriding influence on this sensation.

Optical illusions give rise not only to errors in relation to the horizontal plane, i.e. errors in the height estimation but also in relation to the true vertical plane, i.e. in the estimation of the horizontal distance from the landmark. Imaginary horizontal distances may also be determined by a sinusoid; they are proportional to distance D of landmark and to sine of angle ($a + \theta$). It seems that imaginary horizontal distances are not as hazardous as imaginary heights; nevertheless they also lead the pilot to wrong reaction.

My Conclusions

In endeavoring to analyze the errors that occur with respect to the three axes of an airplane, I have arrived at the following conclusions: —

1. With respect to the directional axis:
No error seems possible when the specific landmark viewed by the pilot in one direction cannot be seen in another direction.

2. With respect to the rolling axis: —
A pilot sitting in the left-hand seat and looking to his left: —
a) The illusion of flying.horizontally when he is flying inclined to the right is dangerous because he believes himself to be higher than he really is and, furthermore, the airplane is flying in an abnormal attitude.
b) Illusion of horizontal flight when he is flying inclined to the left does not seem dangerous. As a matter of fact, in approaching the ground, the visual stimuli automatically correct such an abnormal situation. For pilots in the right hand seat looking towards the right, the same phenomena are obtained but in an inverse sense.

3. With respect to the pitching axis: —
a) The illusion of flying horizontally with respect to a landmark when flying more nose-

up than imagined is dangerous because the pilot believes himself to be higher than he really is. The angle at which a pilot observes a point of light on the horizon depends on his altitude and his distance from the point. Evaluation of that angle is not a matter of mathematics but is one of feeling (purely subjective). This illusion may have serious consequences. In fact, if the pilot without realizing it changes the angle of his airplane with respect to its initial position by as little as one degree, this error translates into differences in altitude of:

17.5 meters for a landmark 1 kilometer away
35.0 meters at 2 kilometers away
87.5 meters for a landmark 5 kilometers away
175.0 meters for a landmark 10 kilometers away

The illusion cited above must certainly be the cause of many aircraft accidents occurring just before the airplane reaches the airfield, especially when no adequate landmark can be found in the approaches (for example: an airdrome located on the edge of the ocean).
b) The illusion of horizontal flight when the aircraft is actually nose-down does not seem dangerous because this attitude will be automatically corrected before the airplane reaches the ground.

FIG. 12.   ILLUSION ABOVE A LINE OF LIGHTS OR LANDMARKS

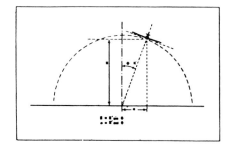

So far I've limited myself to describing illusions which occur when the trajectory of the aircraft corresponds to one or the other of the three axes of freedom of the airplane taken singly, but I find it more difficult to analyze the illusions and their effect with respect to the three axes when taken simultaneously. However, these are complex illusions which can be dangerous and are of frequent occurrence, especially in final approach. Therein lies a vast field of study in which the results can contribute very greatly to improvement in aviation safety. In my opinion, here are the things which must be done to avoid accidents due to illusions:-

1. *A most comprehensive study of the different phenomena of illusions and their consequences.*
2. *Take effective steps to make flight personnel aware of the danger of illusions.*
3. *Improvement in method of flight as follows:-*
   Until now at least a part of every flight, the landing, was made under visual contact conditions. It is at this part of the flight that illusions may loom up. It is therefore necessary to reduce the duration of this visual contact phase to a minimum by flight on instruments (as long as possible). It is of the utmost importance that the duration of the transition period from instrument flight to visual contact flight be as short as possible in order to avoid the possibility of the creation of illusions. The optimum point of transition would seem to be at the passage of the middle marker on the I.L.S. system which is usually found at a distance of 3,500 feet plus or minus 500 feet from the set down point. It is about this distance away that the first approach lights should be located. In the case of landing by G.C.A. the transition point is about 400 meters from the end of the landing strip in service. In this case the pilot of an airplane flying at 600 meters a second has only about 6 seconds and the view of two transverse bars in the approach light system of Calvert to adapt himself to contact conditions before touching down. In my opinion it would be interesting to determine if this is sufficient time for pilots subject to optical illusions to make the necessary corrections.
   It is obvious that automatic systems of flight when they work without failure and without the intervention of the pilot in flying the airplane should eliminate entirely any possibility of false maneuver due to sensory illusion.
4. *Improvement in radio aid to allow the pilot to determine exactly the transition point from instrument flight to contact flight.*
5. *Improvement of visual aids in the approach sector to give the pilot instantly his exact position under contact flight whether by day or by night.*

Psychology defines certain laws concerning the recognition of objects based on differences between the configuration and their background. Certain char-

acteristics by which they may be differentiated may be defined by:

1. *Form of the structure*
2. *Contours*
3. *Characteristics of a comparable object*
4. *The tendency to stand out from the background*
5. *Color differentiation*
6. *Stability of form*

These are the properties, therefore, which should produce visual stimuli to permit the recognition of an object. They are more marked in the daytime even in poor visibility than they are at night. In fact, at night the surface of the earth loses all its characteristics which yield exact information, and observation on the ground will not furnish adequate stimulus for recognition, location, etc.

It has long been since recognized that a system of lights is necessary to reconstruct landmarks artificially to permit the pilot to make normal landings. The approach lights of the Calvert system are those, in my opinion, which reproduce best the conditions of stimuli which have been laid out above. As a matter of fact, in this system the determination of position with respect to the directional axis and the axis of roll does not present any ambiguity whatever, a condition which is absolutely necessary to avoid illusions. At the same time the position with respect to the pitching axis and a knowledge of altitude may be easily deduced by direct observation of the lights.

Finally, in flying down the central axis of the Calvert system, the pilot steers to a fixed line of lights which are flashing by underneath his plane, while on a system of bi-lineal lights he steers between the rows of lights which are flashing on each side. This condition makes the steering more difficult, especially if the visibility is very low, because the pilot cannot imagine as easily the picture of his exact position.

This is, therefore, the system which, combined with adequate radio landing aid, permits, in my opinion, safe landing conditions of visibility of 300 meters and even of 200 meters for well trained pilots.

(From Captain Cocquyt's 1950 paper published by FSF.)

The human element is always responsible for these accidents. If these could always be foreseen, he would naturally take adequate measures to prevent their occurrence. As far as sensory illusions are concerned, these measures must be generally varied and complex, whereas the optical illusions of the pilot may be eliminated by taking account of a sensation exclusively when it is duplicated by instrument readings. It is imperative to warn all pilots against such illusions. To this end it would be necessary to devote more time to the study of the problem and to disseminate reports covering this question. In my opinion however, the best means would be to produce a film presenting some illusions of current life, the illusions to which one may be subject in flight, and statistical data of the accidents resulting from these illusions, stressing their importance. I am naturally unable to produce such a film myself and even less able to carry out a thorough study of the human element. The authorities responsible for this task would, in performing it, bring a further contribution to the realm of flight safety.

LOST HORIZONS

The following article was authored by Col. H. G. Moseley, Chief, Aero Medical Safety Division, Directorate of Flight Safety Research, and reprinted from Flying Safety Magazine.

RECENTLY AN ELEMENT of two fighter aircraft was making an instrument approach to a strange airfield. It was night and very dark. The element leader let down to 3500 feet and was in a 30-degree bank onto final approach when he suddenly became quite confused as to his direction. He immediately brought his aircraft back to level flight, regained his sense of direction and again kicked into the 30-degree bank to complete the turn onto final. At this point he was surprised to find his cockpit illuminated by a bright flash of light behind and below him.

That flash was caused by wingman's aircraft when it struck the ground and exploded. Result—scratch one wingman.

No one ever knew exactly what happened, and lacking final proof, it might eventually have been relegated to the limbo of "Cause Undetermined Accidents." The evidence in this case, however, pointed straight to one of the most vicious killers that is free in the skies today.

This enemy—this annihilator of pilots and crews—is all the more dangerous because of the pseudonyms and aliases by which it is identified. Generally, it is termed as *Vertigo*. It is also called "Spatial Disorientation" and sometimes identified as "The Leans." Some survivors have simply stated that they were attacked by "Monumental Confusion." But no matter what you term it—and for simplicity we will call it Vertigo—it is a good thing to become acquainted with. And if you are a pilot, you'd better know all about it; know what it is like, what brings it on and how to avoid it. This is fundamental if you want to survive.

To understand Vertigo, one must understand a little about three of man's special senses: sense of vision, of pressure and equilibrium. The latter two demand most of our attention because it is upon them that vertigo preys. These senses of pressure and equilibrium are quite remarkable. Without them we would be completely helpless as soon as darkness sets in. If we did not have these phenomena which give us information about our position and direction, we could only move about in daylight. As it is, however, we can walk in complete darkness or even bend or turn and progress to distant points in an upright and balanced position.

The sense of pressure lies within our muscles, skin and to some extent within our joints, and tells us the direction of the force of gravity. In other words when we stand, the pressure we feel on the soles of our feet and within our legs tells us that our feet are on firm ground and that we are standing upright. And no matter what position we are in, these pressure senses tell us the direction of up and down. In some diseases where these senses of pressure are destroyed, the individual has to be led by hand when it is dark, otherwise he would stumble, fall and be unable to right himself again.

Our sense of equilibrium is even more remarkable. It is governed by what is called our vestibular apparatus. These are small special organs which are constructed a good deal like a set of gyros and are set within our skulls, one within the bones by either ear. (Fig. 1.) These human gyros are filled with fluid. When we turn, the fluid lags a bit like water in a wine glass when you twirl the stem. We are able to feel this lag and it tells us we are turning. Similarly when we stop turning, the fluid which by now has started to move continues to flow for a moment. This is quite important because as you turn rapidly the flow in the vestibular gyros gets to moving rapidly too; and when you stop suddenly this continued flow of fluid makes you feel strange. It may make you dizzy, and it may make it very difficult to walk straight. Every child who has wound himself up in a swing, unwound rapidly and then tried to walk, can tell you about these sensations. Such dizziness caused by the too rapid movement of fluid in our vestibular gyros is a tremendous factor in the cause of vertigo.

This would be of interest but of no great importance if we remained on the ground. Very few pedestrians or sleep walkers get into trouble because of their senses of equilibrium. In flying, however, the senses of pressure and equilibrium are subjected to strange and unusual compromises. They can become so misled and so confused that they give the pilot completely erroneous information concerning his direction or orientation. Hence, the term *disorientation.*

Consider first of all the simple sense of pressure which we feel with our skin, muscles and joints, and which tells us which end is up. These senses simply measure gravity and as gravity pushes down, where we feel the most pressure must be straight down. However, almost the only type of gravity which man has known from time immemorial has been the gravitational pull of the earth, and therefore man has been conditioned to believe that the greatest gravitational pull must be straight down toward the center of the earth.

But in flying, one continually changes the direction of gravity. If we turn the aircraft and hold it in a turn the greatest degree of gravity is directed toward the periphery of the circular plane we are establishing, and here is where our senses of pressure get confused. To these senses, the greatest pressure we feel should be straight down, not sideways, and

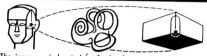

The inner ear is located in the head approximately as shown and is about the size of the black dot.

Each canal and the common sac is completely filled with fluid. Into the ends of each canal, project small sensory hairs which are deflected by any movement of the fluid in the canal, and which are responsible for the sensation of turning in any of the three planes or vectors thereof.

As the head is rotated, the canal in that plane of rotation will move with respect to the fluid in it. Since this fluid has inertia, the resulting deflection of the sensory hairs will cause a sensation of turning.

Enlarged, the actual structure is similar to drawing. The semicircular canals are circular tubes lying at right angles to each other in the planes shown.

The static organ is located in the bottom part of the common sac, and consists of delicate sensory hairs projecting upward, on which rest small crystals.

The load borne by these sensory hairs changes in the head with every change of the head with respect to gravity, and this creates the sensation of tilting the head or body.

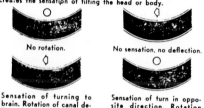

No rotation.   No sensation, no deflection.

Sensation of turning to brain. Rotation of canal deflects hairs.   Sensation of turn in opposite direction. Rotation stopped deflects hairs in opposite direction.

Sensation of movement to brain.

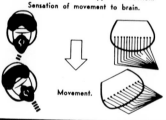

Movement.

FIGURE ONE

our brain receives a continuing series of messages telling us we are sitting straight up and down, exactly like we would be in a chair within our home. If we close our eyes while in such a turn, or if it is dark or cloudy, we can not help but believe these messages, and when we open them again and see that we are really in a 90-degree bank, it is difficult to believe our eyes.

In fact, there was one accident not long ago where two pilots flying jet fighters at 30,000 feet at night became separated in a cloud. When they emerged, one pilot noticed the other aircraft upside down above him. It was only subsequent to the accident when he compared notes with this other pilot that he finally realized that it was he himself who had been upside down. This all happened because he inadvertently rolled through the cloud and heeded only the gravitational pressure that continued to press on

the seat of his pants. He admitted that his instruments were acting strangely.

However, it is the vestibular gyros which can confuse us most of all. When we turn or roll or whirl or otherwise agitate the fluid in these gyros, the messages our brain receives become most garbled. And hence the rest of the story of the upside down pilot we just mentioned. When he fell out of his unnatural position, he was thrown into a spin, and although he brought the aircraft out of the spin on several occasions, he immediately went into another spin. Finally noticing the altimeter unwinding at an alarming rate, he decided, with considerable justification, to leave his topsy-turvy aircraft which appeared to be bent on his destruction.

But, it was not the aircraft which was trying to destroy him. In fact, the aircraft was functioning properly and only responding to the unreasonable kicks and thrusts he was delivering to the stick and rudder. What was bent upon his destruction was our old acquaintance Vertigo. In this case the pilot first became confused through his sense of pressure, but when the fluid in his vestibular gyros began to whirl he was thrown into a series of overpowering and false sensations. When he would come out of a spin his organs of equilibrium would tell him that he was still spinning but in the other direction, and in trying to correct for this, he would spin again, and so on ad infinitum. He was truly a victim of "monumental confusion."

However, one does not have to spin an airplane to get vertigo. Even turns, dives and climbs, if they are sharp enough or prolonged enough, can stimulate our sense of equilibrium to a degree where we may become confused. And here lies another consideration of utmost importance. Our vestibular gyros are not simple little organs. On the contrary, they are remarkably well constructed and are able to pick up several different sensations. For example, they sense turns to the right or left, feel movements of up or down or back and forth, and even respond to the sensation of dropping. In other words, they tell us whether we are turning, twirling, somersaulting, slithering or falling. It is quite possible to stimulate several of these varying planes of our vestibular apparatus at the same time. And this can lead to rather tragic results.

About a year and a half ago FLYING SAFETY published an article concerning pilots who dove their fighter or interceptor aircraft into the ground immediately after attempting to change UHF radio channels. In this maneuver, they had to turn their heads to the right and look down toward the rear of the right console. If their aircraft was also in a bank when they turned their heads so sharply, they started the fluid moving in several planes of their vestibular apparatus. Then when they looked forward again their senses were so severely compromised that they were actually incapacitated for a few seconds. If you do not believe this is possible, just sit on a piano stool, turn your head sharply to one side or simply tilt it back about 60 degrees, then have a friend twirl the stool around about five times in ten seconds while your head is still sideways or backwards. After the fifth turn, stop suddenly and bring your head sharply forward. Many people who have tried this have actually and involuntarily thrown themselves sideward off the stool. If you were trying to fly an aircraft at this time, you would find yourself completely incapacitated.

Having the head turned or tilted forward or back while the aircraft is in a sharp bank is probably one of the worst situations a flyer can put himself into. This indicates that it is quite important to keep your head straight and level while you are in a sharp turn, otherwise you will start so many of your vestibular gyros twirling that confusion is almost inevitable.

However, all pilots who fly will encounter various sensations which arise from the unusual stresses and strains which flying puts upon their senses of pressure and equilibrium. Major General Harry G. Armstrong, in his book "Principles and Practices of Aviation Medicine" describes the following false sensations of flight. They are of tremendous importance.

● *Unperceived Motion.* The organs of equilibrium are fairly insensitive to gradual changes of direction, so that in blind flight there may be motions of the airplane which are not sensed. The average person can be tilted about 10.6 degrees downward or 24 degrees upward without being aware of any change. Also, the body must be rotated with an acceleration of more than about two degrees per second before such motion is sensed. As a consequence in blind flight the airplane might dive or climb at a fairly steep angle and bank or turn at a fairly high rate without there being any sensation of any change from straight and level flight.

● *Sensation of Climbing While Turning.* In a fairly sharp horizontal turn the banking of the airplane is not usually sensed, but there is an awareness of the body being pressed more firmly into the seat as a result of the centrifugal force. As a consequence, the sensation is that of a zoom upward, and is interpreted as such, and the natural reaction is to push forward on the stick.

● *Sensation of Diving During Recovery from a Turn.* During recovery from a turn, the pressure of the body on the seat is decreased which results in a sensation similar to that when the airplane is nosed over from level flight into a dive. As a consequence, in blind flight return to level flight creates the false sensation of diving, causing a tendency to pull back on the control column and resulting in a steep climb and possible stall.

● *Estimating the Degree of Bank.* Because the amount of bank of an airplane, in going into a turn, is below the threshold of the organs of equilibrium, the degree of bank attained during blind flying is usually underestimated. This causes the pilot to bank too steeply in going into a turn, and to over-correct in a return to level flight which results in a bank in the opposite direction.

● *Unperceived Banks.* Under ordinary circumstances, if one tilts the body sideways, this can be easily sensed since the pull of gravity on the body makes us aware of this tilt. In an aircraft turn such a sensation of tilting does not exist because the body is acted upon not only by gravity but by centrifugal force and the resultant of these two forces acts in a line perpendicular, not to the earth, but to the transverse axis of the airplane which creates a sensation of sitting erect.

● *Sensation of Opposite Tilt in a Skid.* If an airplane skids during a turn, the centrifugal force on the body no longer acts perpendicular to the transverse axis of the airplane, and there is a sensation that the airplane is banked in the opposite direction from its true position.

● *Optical Illusions from Clouds.* When flying between cloud layers which are not exactly horizontal, the clouds are used as a horizon and the airplane is flown at a corresponding tilt away from its true level attitude.

● *Sensation of Diving Beyond the Vertical.* If in a very sharp turn or in a spin, the head is suddenly turned downward, as might occur from looking at an object on the floor of the cockpit, the vestibular apparatus of the inner ear is acted upon by two distinct rotary motions at the same time, with the result that there is a sensation of falling forward. Thus, the airplane feels as though it had suddenly nosed downward beyond the vertical, and the natural response of the pilot is to pull back on the control column which, in a spin, only aggravates the situation.

This type of motion, i.e., when an active movement of the head is made in a plane at right angles to a plane of passive rotation, is known as Coriolis acceleration. This may take place, for example, during a spin if the pilot should meanwhile move his head up or down. If the head is moved (turned) downward during a left hand spin, the resultant sensation is of rotation to the left and downward and the falling reaction is to the right and downward. When present, the Coriolis reaction usually produces marked vertigo and is especially dangerous in aviation for that reason.

● *Sensation of Reversal of Rotation.* If, in blind flight, any rotary motion persists for a short time and is then either retarded or stopped, the fluid in the affected semicircular canal continues to rotate and creates a sensation of rotation in the opposite direction. Thus, after a recovery from a spin to the left, there is then a sensation of turning to the right, which the pilot attempts to correct and thereby causes the airplane to spin again to the left.

In view of such compromises, one might well ask, "What can a poor pilot do?" Fortunately, Vertigo—though a ruthless deceiver—can be shaken off when it first attacks, providing you muster enough resolve to ignore its false messages. And this means believing your instruments more than you believe your senses.

X-661

To quote again from General Armstrong. "Most of the time spent in learning instrument flying is nothing more or less than learning to ignore the false sensations from the organs of equilibrium. No one ever learns instrument flying who has not been thoroughly convinced that the sensations are always wrong when they disagree with the instruments."

However, when Vertigo strikes hard it may be almost impossible to ignore the confusing messages that our brain is receiving. Thus, it is best to avoid Vertigo insofar as possible. Here are a few simple points that will give you reasonable immunity:

● Always remember that your instruments are more reliable than your sensations.

● Know the false sensations of flight and be ready to identify them.

● Instrument flight is one condition where it pays to have your head "up and locked." The more you look around the more likely you are to tumble your vestibular gyros.

● Lastly, and most important of all, keep ahead of your instruments. If you can eliminate surprise, you can pretty well eliminate attack. However, once you lose your horizons, be they real or artificial, you are in for a running battle with a most treacherous adversary. And this is one battle you cannot afford to lose.

TAKE-OFF ACCIDENTS

Why have airplanes been "piloted" back into the ground after normal take-offs? A report prepared by Dr. John C. Lane, Department of Aviation Medicine, Civil Aviation, Australia, for presentation at Flight Safety Foundation's Ninth Annual Seminar suggests possible clues. Following is a brief of Dr. Lane's report.

During the investigation of a DC-3 take-off accident in Australia (March, 1954), for which no cause was immediately apparent, an observation was made that over a period of eight years there had been six take-off accidents involving the same type aircraft, five of which had occurred at night. Furthermore, all these night take-offs had been under "fully instrument" conditions, no moonlight and no carpet of ground lights. The one take-off accident by day had a mechanical origin, but the cause assigned to the other five had been speculative. In four of the five cases the aircraft took off normally, then lost height and flew into the sea or ground.

Sensory Illusion

In the search for an operational factor which would explain this pattern, a paper by Professor A.R. Collar was discovered. This paper was the result of a study of a series of RAF night take-off accidents during the early 40's. In it, Professor Collar expressed the view, verified by flight tests, that forward acceleration of an aircraft after take-off causes a sensation of nose-up tilt because the pilot cannot distinguish between the direction of gravity and the resultant of gravity and aircraft acceleration. If the pilot is not fully on instruments, the professor stated, this can induce him to lower the nose, the acceleration in the resulting dive perpetuating the illusion. Literally, the aircraft can enter a shallow dive, with or without turning, and the pilot still will experience the sensation of a steady climb.

Although this illusion was given some publicity about 12 years ago, in the intervening years it seems to have been entirely forgotten. Certainly, it never became part of any formal flying manual available in Australia.

No Horizon

For angles up to 10° this illusory displacement of the vertical under linear acceleration is only manifest when there is no visual information available as to pitch attitude. On visual take-offs, this information

is given by the horizon; on non-visual take-offs, by the artificial horizon. When the atmosphere is clear, however, the pilot may be tempted to forsake his artificial horizon and look outside.

If it is very dark and the direction of take-off is away from built-up areas, there is nothing to be seen which can give horizon reference, and so the pilot is apt to get this false impression of the aircraft in pitch attitude. Because it is too dark to see the ground, loss of height or altitude is not apparent. The magnitude of this apparent displacement is not small. Although made for another purpose, measurements of the acceleration of transport aircraft just after take-off gave values of 5° or more for the apparent tilt.

Review of records shows that take-off accidents of this kind are not uncommon. A fairly recent example occurred at Shannon, Ireland in 1954. There was no moon at the time and the direction of take-off is understood to have been away from built-up areas. The crew reported the take-off to be normal almost until the moment the aircraft struck the water. The report of the inquiry gives an estimated flight path with a maximum altitude of 170 feet. At this point there was a nose-down change of pitch due to flap retraction and the aircraft thereafter lost height. It was accelerating throughout the whole of the 39 seconds of flight. The report gave as a main cause:

"Failure of the Captain to properly correlate and interpret his instrument indications during flap retraction, resulting in the necessary action not being taken in sufficient time."

The average acceleration over the whole flight was about 1/19G, but because of the lag between acceleration and the sensation of tilt, it may be more correct to consider the initial acceleration of 1/14G. The apparent nose-down tilts corresponding to 1/19G and 1/14G are 3° and 4° respectively, thus bracketing the value of 3½° of nose-down change in attitude. It was failure to correct this nose-down change which caused the aircraft's flight path to become a descent. Therefore, this illusion provides a plausible mechanism for the main cause quoted above.

* Reprinted from FSF's Accident Prevention Bulletin 58-1

FAA AC   ·3

X-1191

NTSB Field Offices

Appendix 8 lists the National Transportation Safety Board Field Offices with their addresses and phone numbers. The reasons for contacting the National Transportation Safety Board Field Offices are explained in Chapters I and V.

NTSB FIELD OFFICES

Anchorage, Alaska—Rm. 454, 632 Sixth Ave., Zip Code 99501, Phone (907) 277-0593

Los Angeles, Calif.—8939 South Sepulveda Blvd., Suite 426, Zip Code 90045, Phone (213) 536-6584

Oakland, Calif.—333 Hegenberger Rd., Zip Code 94621, Phone (415) 568-1290

Aurora, Colo.—10255 East 25th Ave., Zip Code 80010, Phone (303) 837-4492

Washington, D.C.—P.O. Box 17226, Gateway Bldg. #1, Dulles Int'l. Airport, Zip Code 20041, Phone (703) 471-1200

Miami Springs, Fla.—4471 N.W. 36th St., Zip Code 33166, Phone (305) 526-2940

Atlanta, Ga.—1720 Peachtree St., N.W., Zip Code 30309, Phone (404) 881-7385

Des Plaines, Ill.—2300 E. Devon Ave., Rm. 140, Zip Code 60018, Phone (312) 827-8858

Kansas City, Mo.—Federal Bldg., Rm. 1443, 601 East 12th St., Zip Code 64106, Phone (816) 374-3576

Jamaica, N.Y.—Federal Bldg., Rm. 102, John F. Kennedy Intl. Airport, Zip Code 11430, Phone (212) 995-3716

Fort Worth, Tex.—Federal Bldg., Rm. 7A07, 819 Taylor St., Zip Code 76102, Phone (817) 334-2616

Seattle, Wash.—19415 Pacific Highway South, Zip Code 98188, Phone (206) 764-3782

National Transportation Accident Investigation School—Gateway Bldg. #1, Dulles Int'l. Airport, P.O. Box 170, Washington, D.C. 20041, Phone (703) 471-1268

FAA REGioNAl
FiEld OfficES

Appendix 9 lists each FAA regional field office with its director, address, phone number, and duty hours. The FAA regional and district offices are good sources of information when questions arise as well as the source of information for the medical films noted in Appendix 2.

DOMESTIC FAA REGIONAL OFFICES

Alaskan Region—Anchorage

Governing Alaska and Aleutian Islands
Lyle K. Brown, Director; 632 Sixth Ave., Anchorage 99501; Phone (907) 265-4201; Duty Officer (907) 262-8112
Areas and Area Coordinators
Anchorage—Frank Babiak, Coordinator; 4510 International Airport Rd., Anchorage 99502; Phone (907) 272-1020
Fairbanks Central Sector—Paul Gallagher, Coordinator; 5460 Airport Way, Fairbanks 99701; Phone (907) 456-4600
Fairbanks North Sector—Thor Weatherby, Coordinator; 5460 Airport Way, Fairbanks 99701; Phone (907) 452-1257

Juneau—Lyndol Pruitt, Coordinator; P.O. Box 1647, Juneau 99801; Phone (907) 586-7245
King Salmon—Carl Fundeen, Coordinator; P.O. Box 67, King Salmon 99613; Phone (907) 246-3321

Central Region—Kansas City

Governing Iowa, Kansas, Missouri, Nebraska
C. R. Melugin, Director; 601 East 12th St., Kansas City, Mo. 64106; Phone (816) 374-5626; Duty Officer (816) 374-3246; Duty Hours 7:30-4:00 (8:30-5:00 EST)

Eastern Region—New York

Governing Delaware, District of Columbia, Maryland, New Jersey, New York, Pennsylvania, Virginia, West Virginia
William E. Morgan, Director; John F. Kennedy Intl. Airport, Jamaica, N.Y. 11430; Phone (212) 995-2801; Duty Officer (212) 995-8555; Duty hours 8:00-4:30 EST (Daylight Saving Time from last Sunday in April through last Sunday in October)

Great Lakes Region—Chicago

Governing Illinois, Indiana, Minnesota, Michigan, Ohio, Wisconsin
John M. Cyrocki, Director; 2300 E. Devon Ave., Des Plaines, Ill. 60018; Phone (312) 694-4500; Duty Officer (312) 694-4401

New England Region—Boston

Governing Connecticut, Maine, Massachusetts, New Hampshire, Rhode Island, Vermont
Robert E. Whittington, Director; 12 New England Executive Park, Burlington, Mass. 01803; Phone Director (617) 273-7244; Duty Officer (617) 273-7000

Northwest Region—Seattle

Governing Idaho, Oregon, Washington
Christian B. Walk, Jr., Director: FAA Building, Boeing Field, King County Int'l., Seattle, Wash. 98108; Phone (206) 767-2780; Duty Officer (206) 767-2600

Pacific Region—Honolulu

Governing Hawaii, Western Pacific
Robert O. Ziegler, Director; P.O. Box 4009, Honolulu, Hawaii 96813; Phone (808) 546-8641; Duty Officer (808) 546-7544

Rocky Mountain Region—Denver

Governing Colorado, Montana, North Dakota, South Dakota, Utah, Wyoming
Mervyn Martin, Director; 10455 East 25th Ave., Aurora, Colo. 80010; Phone (303) 837-3646; Duty Officer (303) 837-4677

Southern Region—Atlanta

Governing Alabama, Florida, Georgia, Mississippi, North Carolina, South Carolina, Tennessee, Kentucky, Puerto Rico, U.S. Virgin Isl., Canal Zone
Phillip M. Swatek, Director; P.O. Box 20636, Atlanta, Ga. 30320; Phone (404) 763-7222; Duty Officer (404) 763-7541; Duty hours 8:30-5 EST

Southwest Region—Fort Worth

Governing Arkansas, Louisiana, New Mexico, Oklahoma, Texas
Henry L. Newman, Director; P.O. Box 1689, Fort Worth, Tex. 76101; Phone (817) 624-4911 ext. 200; Duty Officer (817) 624-4911 ext. 321; Duty hours 8:30-5 (9:30-6 EST)

Western Region—Los Angeles

Governing Arizona, California, Nevada
Leon C. Daugherty (acting), Director; P.O. Box 92007, World Way Postal Center, Los Angeles, Calif. 90009; Phone (213) 536-6427; Duty Officer (213) 536-6435; Duty hours 7:30-4:00 (10:30-7:00 EST)

FAA GENERAL AVIATION DISTRICT OFFICES

Unless otherwise noted, address correspondence to General Aviation District Office, Federal Aviation Administration.

Alaskan Region

Anchorage, Alaska—1515 East 13th Ave., Zip Code 99501; Phone (907) 272-1324, 265-4657, and 265-4673

Fairbanks, Alaska—(Flight Standards District Office), 3788 University Avenue, Zip Code 99701; Phone (907) 452-1276

Juneau, Alaska—(Flight Standards District Office), Juneau Municipal Airport, P.O. Box 2118, Zip Code 99803; Phone (907) 789-0231/2

Central Region

Des Moines, Ia.—3021 Army Post Rd., Zip Code 50321; Phone (515) 284-4094

Kansas City, Kan.—Administration Bldg., 2nd Floor, Fairfax Municipal Airport, Zip Code 66115; Phone (913) 281-3491

Wichita, Kan.—Flight Standards Bldg., Mid-Continent Airport, Zip Code 67209; Phone (316) 943-3244

St. Louis, Mo.—(Flight Standards District Office), 9275 Genaire Dr., Berkeley, Mo. Zip Code 63134; Phone (314) 425-7102

Lincoln, Neb.—General Aviation Bldg. Lincoln Municipal Airport, Zip Code 68524; Phone (402) 471-5485

Eastern Region

Washington, D.C.—(Flight Standards District Office), West Bldg., Room 152, National Airport, Zip Code 20001; Phone (202) 628-1555

Baltimore, Md.—Baltimore-Washington Intl. Airport, Zip Code 21240; Phone (301) 761-2610

Teterboro, N.J.—150 Riser Rd., Teterboro Airport, Zip Code 07608; Phone (201) 288-1745

Albany, N.Y.—Albany County Airport, Zip Code 12211; Phone (518) 869-8482

Farmingdale, N.Y.—Bldg. 53, Republic Airport, Zip Code 11735; Phone (516) 691-3100

Rochester, N.Y.—(Flight Standards District Office), Rochester-Monroe County Airport, Zip Code 14624; Phone (716) 263-5880

Allentown, Pa.—Allentown-Bethlehem-Easton Airport, Zip Code 18103; Phone (215) 264-2888

New Cumberland, Pa.—Capital City Airport, Room 201, Administration Bldg., Zip Code 17070, Phone (717) 782-4528

Philadelphia, Pa.—North Philadelphia Airport, 1st Floor, Administration Bldg., Zip Code 19114; Phone (215) 597-9708

Pittsburgh, Pa.—Allegheny County Airport, West Mifflin, Pa. 15122; Phone (412) 461-7800 and 462-5507

Richmond, Va.—Byrd Field, Sandston, Va. 23150; Phone (804) 222-7494

Charleston, W. Va.—Kanawha Airport, Zip Code 25311; Phone (304) 343-4689

Great Lakes Region

Chicago, Ill.—Box H, DuPage County Airport, West Chicago, Ill. Zip Code 60185; Phone (312) 584-4490

Springfield, Ill.—Box 3, RR #2, Capital Airport, Zip Code 62707; Phone (217) 525-4238

Indianapolis, Ind.—FAA Bldg. #1, Box 41525, Indianapolis International Airport, Zip Code 46241; Phone (317) 247-2491

South Bend, Ind.—1843 Commerce Dr., Zip Code 46628; Phone (219) 232-5843

Detroit, Mich.—Flight Standards Bldg., Willow Run Airport, Ypsilanti, Mich. 48197; Phone (313) 485-2250

Grand Rapids, Mich.—5500 44th St. S.E., Kent County Airport, Zip Code 49508; Phone (616) 456-2427

Minneapolis, Minn.—6201 34th Ave. South, Zip Code 55450; Phone (612)725-3341

Cincinnati, Ohio—Lunken Executive Bldg., 4242 Airport Rd., Zip Code 45226; Phone (513) 684-2183

Cleveland, Ohio—Federal Office Bldg., Cleveland-Hopkins International Airport, Zip Code 44135; Phone (216) 267-0220

Columbus, Ohio—4393 E. 17th Ave., Port Columbus International Airport, Zip Code 43219; Phone (619) 469-7476

Milwaukee, Wisc.—General Mitchell Field, Zip Code 53207; Phone (414) 747-5531

New England Region

Portland, Me.—Portland International Jetport, Zip Code 04102; Phone (207) 774-4484

Boston, Mass.—Norwood Municipal Airport, Norwood, Mass. 02062; Phone (617) 762-2436

Westfield, Mass.—P.O. Box 544, Zip Code 01085; Phone (413) 568-3121

Northwest Region

Boise, Ida.—3113 Airport Way, Zip Code 83705; Phone (208) 384-1238

Eugene, Ore.—Mahlon-Sweet Airport, 90606 Greenhill Rd., Zip Code 97402; Phone (503) 688-9721

Portland, Ore.—Portland-Hillsboro Airport, 3355 N.E. Cornell Rd., Hillsboro, Ore. 97123; Phone (503) 221-2104

Seattle, Wash.—(Flight Standards District Office), FAA Bldg., Boeing Field, Zip Code 98108; Phone (206) 767-2747/2570

Spokane, Wash.—5629 E. Rutter Avenue; Zip Code 99206; Phone (509) 456-4618

Pacific Region

Honolulu, Hawaii—(Flight Standards District Office), P.O. Box 29728; Zip Code 96820; Phone 847-0615

Rocky Mountain Region

Denver, Colo.—Jefferson County Airport, Bldg. 1, Broomfield, Colo. 80020; Phone (303) 466-7326

Billings, Mont.—Room 216, Administration Bldg., Billings Logan International Airport; Code 59101; Phone (406) 245-6179

Helena, Mont.—Rm. 3, FAA Bldg., Helena Airport, Zip Code 59601; Phone (406) 449-5270

Fargo, N.D.—State University Station, P.O. Box 5496, Zip Code 58102; Phone (701) 232-8949

Rapid City, S.D.—Regional Airport, R.R. 2, Box 633B, Zip Code 57701; Phone (605) 343-2403

Salt Lake City, Ut.—116 North 2400 West; Zip Code 84116; Phone (801) 524-4247

Casper Wyo.—FAA/WB Bldg., Natrona County Int'l. Airport, Zip Code 82601; Phone (307) 234-8959

Southern Region

Birmingham, Ala.—6500 43rd Ave., North, Zip Code 35206; Phone (205) 254-1393

Jacksonville, Fla.—Craig Field, 855 St. Johns Bluff Rd., Zip Code 32211; Phone (904) 641-7311

Miami, Fla.—Bldg. 121, Opa-Locka Airport, Opa-Locka, Fla. 33054; Phone (305) 681-7431

St. Petersburg, Fla.—St. Petersburg-Clearwater Airport, Zip Code 33520; Phone (813) 531-1434

Atlanta, Ga.—FAA Bldg., Charlie Brown County Airport, Zip Code 30336; Phone (404) 221-6481

Louisville, Ky.—Bowman Field, Zip Code 40205; Phone (502) 582-6116

Jackson, Miss.—P.O. Box 6273, Pearl Branch, Zip Code 39208; Phone (601) 969-4633

Charlotte, N.C.—FAA Bldg., Municipal Airport, P.O. Box 27005, Zip Code 28219; Phone (704) 392-3214

Raleigh, N.C.—Rm. 324 Administration Bldg., Raleigh-Durham Airport, P.O. Box 486A, Zip Code 27560; Phone (919) 755-4240

West Columbia, S.C.—Box 200, Columbia Metropolitan Airport, Zip Code 29169; Phone (803) 765-5931

Memphis, Tenn.—2488 Winchester, Rm. 137, Zip Code 38116; Phone (901) 345-0600

Nashville, Tenn.—(Flight Standards District Office), 322 Knapp Blvd., Rm. 101, Nashville Metropolitan Airport, Zip Code 37217; Phone (615) 251-5661

San Juan, P.R.—(Flight Standards District Office), RFD 1, Box 29A, Loiza Station, Zip Code 00914; Phone (809) 791-5050

Southwest Region

Little Rock, Ark.—FAA/Weather Service Bldg., Rm. 201, Adams Field, Zip Code 72202; Phone (501) 372-3437

New Orleans, La.—Rm. 227, New Orleans Lakefront Airport, Zip Code 70126; Phone (504) 241-2506

Shreveport, La.—Terminal Bldg., Room 137 Shreveport Downtown Airport, Zip Code 71107; Phone (318) 226-5379

Albuquerque, N.M.—P.O. Box 9045, Albuquerque Int'l Airport, Zip Code 87119; Phone (505) 247-0156

Oklahoma City, Okla.—FAA Bldg., Wiley Post Airport, Bethany, Okla. 73008, Phone (405) 789-5220

Tulsa, Okla.—Room 110, General Aviation Terminal, Tulsa Int'l Airport, Zip Code 74115; Phone (918) 835-7619

Midland, Tex.—Terminal Bldg., Rm. 213, Midland-Odessa Regional Air Terminal, P.O. Box 6405, Zip Code 79701; Phone (915) 563-0802

Lafayette, La.—Lafayette Airport, Zip Code 70501; Phone (318) 234-2321

Dallas, Tex.—8032 Air Freight La., Love Field Airport, Zip Code 75235; Phone (214) 357-0142

Corpus Christi, Tex.—Rt. 2, Box 903, Zip Code 78408; Phone (512) 884-9331

El Paso, Tex.—Room 202, FAA Bldg., 6795 Convair Rd., Zip Code 79925; Phone (915) 778-6389

Houston, Tex.—8800 Paul B. Koonce Dr., Rm. 152, Zip Code 77061; Phone (713) 643-6504

Lubbock, Tex.—Rt. 3, Box 51, Zip Code 79401; Phone (806) 762-0335

San Antonio, Tex.—1115 Paul Wilkins Rd., Zip Code 78216; Phone (512) 824-9535

Western Region

Phoenix, Ariz.—(Flight Standards District Office), 15041 North Airport Drive, Scottsdale, Ariz., Zip Code 85260; Phone (602) 261-4763

Fresno, Calif.—Fresno Air Terminal, 2401 North Ashley, Zip Code 93727; Phone (209) 487-5306

Oakland, Calif.—(Flight Standards District Office), L 105 Earhart Road, P.O.

Box 2397, Airport Station, Zip Code 94614; Phone (415) 273-7155

Ontario, Calif.—Ontario International Airport, Zip Code 91761; Phone (714) 984-2411

Sacramento, Calif.—Executive Airport, Zip Code 95822; Phone (916) 440-3169

San Diego, Calif.—3750 John J. Montgomery Drive, Zip Code 92123; Phone (714) 293-5280

San Jose, Calif.—1387 Airport Boulevard, Zip Code 95110; Phone (408) 275-7681

Santa Monica, Calif.—Municipal Airport, 3200 Airport Avenue, Suite 3, Zip Code 90405; Phone (213) 391-6701

Van Nuys, Calif.—7120 Hayvenhurst Avenue, Suite 316, Zip Code 91406; Phone (213) 997-3191

Las Vegas, Nev.—(Flight Standards District Office), 5700-C South Haven, Zip code 89119; Phone (702) 736-0666

Reno, Nev.—Terminal Way, Room 230, Reno International Airport, Zip Code 89502; Phone (702) 784-5321

Long Beach, Calif.—(Flight Standards District Office), 2815 E. Spring Street, Zip code 90806; Phone (213) 426-7135

APPENDIX 10

FAR Part 830

Appendix 10 is Part 830 of the Federal Aviation Regulations. Part 830 relates to the notification and reporting of aircraft accidents or incidents and delineates your responsibilities in detail.

PART 830

RULES PERTAINING TO THE NOTIFICATION AND REPORTING OF AIRCRAFT ACCIDENTS OR INCIDENTS AND OVERDUE AIRCRAFT, AND PRESERVATION OF AIRCRAFT WRECKAGE, MAIL, CARGO, AND RECORDS

Subpart A—General

830.1 Applicability.

This Part contains rules pertaining to:
a. Providing notice of and reporting, aircraft accidents and incidents and certain other occurrences in the operation of aircraft when they involve civil aircraft of the United States wherever they occur, or foreign civil aircraft when such events occur in the United States, its territories or possessions.

b. Preservation of aircraft wreckage, mail, cargo, and records involving all civil aircraft in the United States, its territories or possessions.

830.2 Definitions.

As used in this Part, the following words or phrases are defined as follows:

"Aircraft accident" means an occurrence associated with the operation of an aircraft which takes place between the time any person boards the aircraft with the intention of flight until such time as all such persons have disembarked, in which any person suffers death or serious injury as a result of being in or upon the aircraft or by direct contact with the aircraft or anything attached thereto, or in which the aircraft receives substantial damage.

"Fatal injury" means any injury which results in death within 7 days of the accident.

"Operator" means any person who causes or authorizes the operation of an aircraft, such as the owner, lessee or bailee of an aircraft.

"Serious injury" means any injury which (1) requires hospitalization for more than 48 hours, commencing within

7 days from the date the injury was received; (2) results in a fracture of any bone (except simple fractures of fingers, toes or nose); (3) involves lacerations which cause severe hemorrhages, nerve, muscle or tendon damage; (4) involves injury to any internal organ; or (5) involves second- or third-degree burns, or any burns affecting more than 5 percent of the body surface.

"Substantial damage":

1. Except as provided in subparagraph (2) of this paragraph, substantial damage means damage or structural failure which adversely affects the structural strength, performance, or flight characteristics of the aircraft, and which would normally require major repair or replacement of the affected component.

2. Engine failure, damage limited to an engine, bent fairings or cowling, dented skin, small puncture holes in the skin or fabric, ground damage to rotor or propeller blades, damage to landing gear, wheels, tires, flaps, engine accessories, brakes, or wing tips are not considered "substantial damage" for the purpose of this Part.

Subpart B—Initial Notification of Aircraft Accidents, Incidents, and Overdue Aircraft

830.5   Immediate Notification.

The operator of an aircraft shall immediately, and by the most expeditious means available, notify the nearest National Transportation Safety Board (Board), field office[1] when:

a. An aircraft accident or any of the following listed incidents occur:

1. Flight control system malfunction or failure;
2. Inability of any required flight crewmember to perform his normal flight duties as a result of injury or illness;
3. Turbine engine rotor failures excluding compressor blades and turbine buckets;
4. In-flight fire; or
5. Aircraft collide in flight.

b. An aircraft is overdue and is believed to have been involved in an accident.

830.6   Information to Be Given in Notification.

The notification required in 830.5 shall contain the following information, if available:

a. Type, nationality, and registration marks of the aircraft;
b. Name of owner, and operator of the aircraft;
c. Name of the pilot-in-command;
d. Date and time of the accident;
e. Last point of departure and point of intended landing of the aircraft;
f. Position of the aircraft with reference to some easily defined geographical point;
g. Number of persons aboard, number killed, and number seriously injured;
h. Nature of the accident, the weather and

----

[1]The National Transportation Safety Board field offices are listed under U.S. Government in the telephone directories in the following cities: Anchorage, Alaska; Chicago, Ill.; Denver, Colo.; Fort Worth, Tex.; Kansas City, Mo.; Los Angeles, Calif.; Miami, Fla.; New York, N.Y.; Oakland, Calif.; Seattle, Wash.; Washington, D.C.

the extent of damage to the aircraft, so far as is known;

i. A description of any explosives, radioactive materials, or other dangerous articles carried.

Subpart C—Preservation of Aircraft Wreckage, Mail, Cargo, and Records

830.10 Preservation of Aircraft Wreckage, Mail, Cargo, and Records.

a. The operator of an aircraft is responsible for preserving to the extent possible any aircraft wreckage, cargo, and mail aboard the aircraft, and all records, including tapes of flight recorders and voice recorders, pertaining to the operation and maintenance of the aircraft and to the airmen involved in an accident or incident for which notification must be given until the Board takes custody thereof or a release is granted pursuant to 831.17.

b. Prior to the time the Board or its authorized representative takes custody of aircraft wreckage, mail, or cargo, such wreckage, mail, or cargo may not be disturbed or moved except to the extent necessary:

1. To remove persons injured or trapped;
2. To protect the wreckage from further damage; or
3. To protect the public from injury.

c. Where it is necessary to disturb or move aircraft wreckage, mail or cargo, sketches, descriptive notes, and photographs shall be made, if possible, of the accident locale including original position and condition of the wreckage and any significant impact marks.

d. The operator of an aircraft involved in an accident or incident, as defined in this Part, shall retain all records and reports, including all internal documents and memoranda dealing with the accident or incident, until authorized by the Board to the contrary.

Subpart D—Reporting of Aircraft Accidents, Incidents, and Overdue Aircraft

830.15 Reports and Statements to Be Filed.

a. **Reports.** The operator of an aircraft shall file a report as provided in paragraph (c) of this section on Board Form 6120.1 or Board Form 6120.2 within 10 days after an accident, or after 7 days if an overdue aircraft is still missing. A report on an incident for which notification is required by 830.5(a) shall be filed only as requested by an authorized representative of the Board.

b. **Crewmember statement.** Each crewmember, if physically able at the time the report is submitted, shall attach thereto a statement setting forth the facts, conditions, and all circumstances relating to the accident or incident as they appear to him to the best of his knowledge and belief. If the crewmember is incapacitated, he shall submit the statement as soon as he is physically able.

c. **Where to file the reports.** The operator of an aircraft shall file with the Field Office of the Board nearest the accident or incident any report required by this section.

Cause/Factor Table—
U.S. General
Aviation Accidents

A listing of cause/factor tables in the United States general aviation accidents for the year 1977 follows. Note that almost all accidents are caused by pilots. Mechanical failures are extremely rare and when implicated, almost always involve the landing gear and/or tires. A word to the wise should be sufficient!

CAUSE/FACTOR TABLE
U.S. GENERAL AVIATION ACCIDENTS ALL OPERATIONS 1977

(Excludes accidents without causal assignment)

Involves 4228 total accidents
Involves   673 fatal accidents

DETAILED CAUSE/FACTOR	FATAL ACCIDENTS		
	CAUSE	FACTOR	TOTAL
Pilot			
Pilot in command			
Attempted operation w/known deficiencies in equipment	7	6	13
Attempted operation beyond experience/ability level	41	16	57
Became lost/disoriented	8	1	9
Continued VFR flight into adverse weather conditions	105	4	109
Continued into known area of severe turbulence	3		3
Delayed action in aborting takeoff			
Delayed in initiating go-around	6	2	8
Diverted attention from operation of aircraft	17	1	18
Exceeded design stress limits of aircraft	31		31
Failed to extend landing gear			
Failed to retract landing gear			
Retracted gear prematurely			
Inadvertently retracted gear			
Failed to see and avoid other aircraft	29		29
Failed to see and avoid objects or obstructions	33		33
Failed to obtain/maintain flying speed	185		185
Misjudged speed, altitude or clearance	3		3
Failed to maintain adequate rotor RPM	5		5
Failed to use or incorrectly used misc equipment	2		2
Failed to follow approved procedures, directives, etc	14	9	23
Improper operation of powerplant & powerplant controls	10	4	14
Improper operation of brakes and/or flight controls			
Improper operation of flight controls	36	2	38
Premature lift off	4		4
Improper level off	1	1	2
Improper IFR operation	20	1	21
Improper in-flight decisions or planning	67	7	74
Improper compensation for wind conditions		1	1
Inadequate preflight preparation and/or planning	72	21	93
Inadequate supervision of flight	9	1	10
Lack of familiarity with aircraft	5	24	29
Mismanagement of fuel	34		34
Exercised poor judgment	29	8	37
Operated carelessly	2		2
Selected unsuitable terrain	5		5
Improper starting procedures			
Started engine without proper assistance/equipment			
Taxied/parked without proper assistance			

NONFATAL ACCIDENTS			ALL ACCIDENTS		
CAUSE	FACTOR	TOTAL	CAUSE	FACTOR	TOTAL
28	9	37	35	15	50
39	16	55	80	32	112
39	8	47	47	9	56
52	6	58	157	10	167
3		3	6		6
46	1	47	46	1	47
97	12	109	103	14	117
64	23	87	81	24	105
3		3	34		34
33		33	33		33
7	1	8	7	1	8
5		5	5		5
17		17	17		17
45	2	47	74	2	76
122	2	124	155	2	157
366	1	367	551	1	552
22		22	25		25
33		33	38		38
4	1	5	6	1	7
48	14	62	62	23	85
92	13	105	102	17	119
170	2	172	170	2	172
86	8	94	122	10	132
41	2	43	45	2	47
206	3	209	207	4	211
10		10	30	1	31
162	9	171	229	16	245
143	9	152	143	10	153
399	48	447	471	69	540
82	6	88	91	7	98
49	73	122	54	97	151
261		261	295		295
43	4	47	72	12	84
1	4	5	3	4	7
200	15	215	205	15	220
3		3	3		3
15	1	16	15	1	16
13		13	13		13

DETAILED CAUSE/FACTOR	FATAL ACCIDENTS		
	CAUSE	FACTOR	TOTAL
Failed to assure the gear was down and locked			
Initiated flight in adverse weather conditions	31	1	32
Control interference	1		1
Spontaneous-improper action			
Misjudged distance, speed, and altitude	10	1	11
Misjudged distance and speed	3		3
Misjudged distance	1		1
Misjudged distance and altitude	6		6
Misjudged speed and altitude			
Misjudged speed			
Misjudged speed and clearance	2		2
Misjudged altitude and clearance	17		17
Misjudged altitude	19		19
Misjudged clearance	13		13
Inadequate training of student			
Misunderstanding of orders or instructions	1		1
Improper recovery from bounced landing		1	1
Incapacitation	9		9
Physical impairment	23	21	44
Spatial disorientation	95		95
Psychological condition	1		1
Misused or failed to use flaps	5	4	9
Failed to maintain directional control	1		1
Selected wrong runway relative to existing wind	2	2	4
Failed to abort takeoff	7		7
Failed to initiate go-around	3		3
Direct entries	1		1
Subtotal	1034	139	1173
Copilot			
Delayed in initiating go-around	1		1
Failed to obtain/maintain flying speed	1		1
Improper operation of powerplant & powerplant controls			
Improper operation of brakes and/or flight controls			
Improper operation of flight controls	1		1
Improper compensation for wind conditions	1		1
Inadequate preflight preparation and/or planning			
Lack of familiarity with aircraft	1	1	2
Mismanagement of fuel			
Failure to relinquish control	1		1
Control interference			
Spontaneous-improper action			
Misjudged distance and altitude			
Misunderstanding of orders or instructions			
Physical impairment	1	1	2
Subtotal	7	2	9

NONFATAL ACCIDENTS			ALL ACCIDENTS		
CAUSE	FACTOR	TOTAL	CAUSE	FACTOR	TOTAL
24		24	24		24
23	3	26	54	4	58
			1		1
10		10	10		10
31	1	32	41	2	43
164	8	172	167	8	175
4		4	5		5
114	4	118	120	4	124
15	2	17	15	2	17
8	2	10	8	2	10
5		5	7		7
29		29	46		46
19		19	38		38
92		92	105		105
2	2	4	2	2	4
3	1	4	4	1	5
112	5	117	112	6	118
2		2	11		11
4	4	8	27	25	52
14		14	109		109
			1		1
27	14	41	32	18	50
280		280	281		281
55	8	63	57	10	67
61	4	65	68	4	72
131	11	142	134	11	145
			1		1
	363	4641	5312	502	5814
			1		1
			1		1
		1	1		1
		2	2		2
			1		1
			1		1
		1	1		1
			1	1	2
		1	1		1
			1		1
		1	1		1
		1	1		1
		2	2		2
		1	1		1
			1	1	2
		10	17	2	19

DETAILED CAUSE/FACTOR	FATAL ACCIDENTS		
	CAUSE	FACTOR	TOTAL
Dual student			
Continued VFR flight into adverse weather conditions			
Delayed action in aborting takeoff			
Delayed in initiating go-around			
Diverted attention from operation of aircraft			
Failed to extend landing gear			
Inadvertently retracted gear			
Failed to see other aircraft			
Failed to see and avoid objects or obstructions			
Failed to obtain/maintain flying speed	4		4
Misjudged distance, speed, altitude or clearance			
Failed to maintain adequate rotor RPM			
Improper operation of powerplant & powerplant controls			
Improper operation of brakes and/or flight controls			
Improper operation of flight controls			
Premature lift-off			
Improper level off			
Improper in-flight decisions or planning			
Improper compensation for wind conditions			
Lack of familiarity with aircraft			
Selected unsuitable terrain			
Failure to relinquish control			
Control interference			
Spontaneous-improper action			
Misjudged distance, speed, and altitude			
Misjudged distance and speed			
Misjudged distance and altitude	1		1
Misjudged speed and altitude			
Misjudged clearance			
Misunderstanding of orders or instructions			
Improper recovery from bounced landing	1		1
Spatial disorientation	1		1
Misused or failed to use flaps			
Failed to maintain directional control			
Failed to abort takeoff			
Failed to initiate go-around			
Subtotal	7		7
Check pilot			
Inadequate supervision of flight			
Subtotal			
Personnel			
Flight instructor			
Inadequate supervision of flight		2	2
Inadequate training of student			

NONFATAL ACCIDENTS			ALL ACCIDENTS		
CAUSE	FACTOR	TOTAL	CAUSE	FACTOR	TOTAL
1		1	1		1
1		1	1		1
1		1	1		1
1		1	1		1
1		1	1		1
2		2	2		2
1		1	1		1
2		2	2		2
6		6	10		10
1		1	1		1
3		3	3		3
2		2	2		2
5		5	5		5
12		12	12		12
1		1	1		1
9		9	9		9
1		1	1		1
5		5	5		5
	1	1		1	1
1		1	1		1
5		5	5		5
4		4	4		4
3		3	3		3
	1	1		1	1
3		3	3		3
12		12	13		13
3		3	3		3
2		2	2		2
2		2	2		2
1		1	2		2
			1		1
2		2	2		2
10		10	10		10
1		1	1		1
3		3	3		3
107	2	109	114	2	116
2	1	3	2	1	3
2	1	3	2	1	3
14	1	15	14	3	17
2	6	8	2	6	8

DETAILED CAUSE/FACTOR	FATAL ACCIDENTS		
	CAUSE	FACTOR	TOTAL
Maintenance, servicing, inspection			
Improper maintenance (maintenance personnel)	4		4
Improper maintenance (owner personnel)	1	1	2
Improperly serviced aircraft (ground crew)		1	1
Improperly serviced aircraft (owner-pilot)			
Inadequate inspection of aircraft (maintenance personnel)	4		4
Inadequate inspection of aircraft (owner-pilot personnel)		1	1
Inadequate maintenance and inspection	10	2	12
Other			
UNK/NR			
Operational supervisory personnel			
Inadequate supervision of flight crew		1	1
Inadequate supervision/training of ramp crews			
Failure to provide adequate directives, manuals, equipment			
Deficiency, company maintained eqmt, serv, regulations		1	1
Weather personnel			
Incorrect weather forecast	1	3	4
Traffic control personnel			
Failure or delay in initiating emergency procedures			
Failure to advise of unsafe weather condition		1	1
Failure to advise of other traffic			
Issued improper or conflicting instructions		1	1
Inadequate spacing of aircraft			
Other		1	1
Airport supervisory personnel			
Improper maintenance-airport facilities			
Failure to notify of unsafe cond/and or failure to mark			
Improper/inadequate snow removal			
Improper inspection of facilities			
Other		1	1
Airways facilities personnel			
Production-design-personnel			
Substandard quality control			
Poor/inadequate design	2	1	3
Other	1		1
Miscellaneous-personnel			
Pilot of other aircraft	30		30
Ground signalman			
Spectator			
Ground crewman	1		1
Passenger	5		5
Driver of vehicle		1	1
Other	1	2	3
Third pilot			
Flight engineer			
Flight personnel			
Flight attendant			

NONFATAL ACCIDENTS			ALL ACCIDENTS		
CAUSE	FACTOR	TOTAL	CAUSE	FACTOR	TOTAL
44	2	46	48	2	50
15	1	16	16	2	18
2	3	5	2	4	6
4		4	4		4
14	2	16	18	2	20
7	3	10	7	4	11
96	18	114	106	20	126
3		3	3		3
2		2	2		2
2		2	2	1	3
1	1	2	1	1	2
4	1	5	4	1	5
6	3	9	6	4	10
			1	3	4
	1	1		1	1
				1	1
	2	2		2	2
3		3	3	1	4
	2	2		2	2
2	1	3	2	2	4
1		1	1		1
3	3	6	3	3	6
7	5	12	7	5	12
1		1	1		1
1		1	1	1	2
1		1	1		1
10	1	11	12	2	14
3		3	4		4
52	3	55	82	3	85
3		3	3		3
2		2	2		2
1	2	3	2	2	4
15	3	18	20	3	23
10	1	11	10	2	12
2	2	4	3	4	7
1		1	1		1

DETAILED CAUSE/FACTOR	FATAL ACCIDENTS		
	CAUSE	FACTOR	TOTAL
Dispatching (air carrier only)			
Subtotal	60	20	80
Airframe			
Wings			
Spars		5	5
Wing attachment fittings, bolts		2	2
Bracing wires, struts			
Skin and attachments	1	2	3
Wingtips			
Other		2	2
Fuselage			
Skin and attachments			
Doors, door frames	1		1
Windshields, widows, canopies			
Seats			
Other		2	2
Landing gear			
Main gear-shock absorbing assy, struts, attachments, etc			
Normal retraction/extension assembly			
Emergency/extension assembly			
Tailwheel assemblies	1		1
Nosewheel assemblies			
Wheels, tires, axles			
Ski assemblies			

NONFATAL ACCIDENTS			ALL ACCIDENTS		
CAUSE	FACTOR	TOTAL	CAUSE	FACTOR	TOTAL
334	67	401	394	87	481
				5	5
1		1	1	2	3
1		1	1		1
			1	2	3
1		1	1		1
				2	2
1	1	2	1	1	2
2	2	4	3	2	5
	1	1		1	1
1		1	1		1
	1	1		3	3
31		31	31		31
24	4	28	24	4	28
7		7	7		7
4	2	6	5	2	7
13		13	13		13
15	8	23	15	8	23
1		1	1		1

CAUSE/FACTOR TABLE
U.S. AIR CARRIERS ALL OPERATIONS 1977

(Excludes 3 accidents with no causal assignments)

Involves 23 total accidents
Involves   4 fatal accidents

DETAILED CAUSE/FACTOR	FATAL ACCIDENTS		
	CAUSE	FACTOR	TOTAL
Pilot			
Pilot in command			
Attempted operation w/known deficiencies in equipment	1		1
Diverted attention from operation of aircraft			
Failed to see and avoid other aircraft			
Failed to see and avoid objects or obstructions			
Failed to follow approved procedures, directives, etc	1		1
Improper IFR operation	1		1
Improper in-flight decisions or planning		1	1
Exercised poor judgment	1		1
Initiated flight in adverse weather conditions			
Misjudged distance, speed, and altitude			
Misjudged clearance			
Failed to maintain directional control			
Direct entries			
Subtotal	4	1	5
Copilot			
Failed to follow approved procedures, directives, etc			
Subtotal			
Personnel			
Flight instructor			
Maintenance, servicing, inspection			
Inadequate maintenance and inspection	1		1
Operational supervisory personnel			
Deficiency, company maintained eqmt, serv, regulations	1		1
Weather personnel			
Traffic control personnel			
Issued improper or conflicting instructions	1		1
Airport supervisory personnel			
Improper maintenance-airport facilities			
Airways facilities personnel			
Production-design-personnel			
Miscellaneous-personnel			
Pilot of other aircraft			
Ground crewman			
Passenger			
Other			
Third pilot			

NONFATAL ACCIDENTS			ALL ACCIDENTS		
CAUSE	FACTOR	TOTAL	CAUSE	FACTOR	TOTAL
			1		1
1		1	1		1
2		2	2		2
1		1	1		1
2		2	3		3
			1		1
				1	1
			1		1
1		1	1		1
1		1	1		1
1		1	1		1
1		1	1		1
1		1	1		1
11		11	15	1	16
1		1	1		1
1		1	1		1
			1		1
			1		1
			1		1
	1	1		1	1
3		3	3		3
1		1	1		1
6		6	6		6
1	1	2	1	1	2

DETAILED CAUSE/FACTOR	FATAL ACCIDENTS		
	CAUSE	FACTOR	TOTAL
Flight engineer			
Flight personnel			
Flight attendant			
Dispatching (air carrier only)			
Failed to keep flight properly advised (flight following)		1	1
Subtotal	3	1	4
Airframe			
Wings			
Fuselage			
Landing gear			
Main gear-shock absorbing assembly, struts, attachments, etc	1		1
Other			
Flight control surfaces			
Subtotal	1		1
Powerplant			

NONFATAL ACCIDENTS			ALL ACCIDENTS		
CAUSE	FACTOR	TOTAL	CAUSE	FACTOR	TOTAL
5		5	5		5
					11
16	2	18	19	3	22
			1		1
	1	1		1	1
	1	1	1	1	2

Survival Manual

Appendix 12 is the search and rescue manual, *Survival* (AFM 64-5), part of which has been deleted. A survival manual should be part of your everyday flight case contents. (Reprinted by permission of U.S.A.F.)

SURVIVAL ON LAND

Immediate Action

GENERAL

- Stay away from the airplane until the engines have cooled and spilled gas has evaporated.
- Check injuries. Give first aid. Make the injured men comfortable. Be careful when removing casualties from the airplane, particularly men with injured backs and fractures.
- Get out of the wind and rain. Throw up a temporary shelter. If you need a fire, start it at once. In cold weather, make hot drinks.
- Get your emergency radio operating on schedule and have other signaling equipment handy.
- Now relax and rest until you are over the shock of the crash. Leave extensive preparations and planning until later.

- After you have rested, organize the camp. Appoint individuals to specific duties. Pool all food and equipment in charge of one man. Prepare a shelter to protect yourself from rain, hot sun, snow, wind, cold, or insects. Collect all possible fuel. Try to have at least a day's stock of fuel on hand. Look for a water supply. Look for animal and plant food.
- Prepare signals so that you will be recognized from the air.
- Start a log book. Include date and cause of crash; probable location; roster of personnel; inventory of food, water, and equipment; weather conditions; and other pertinent data.
- Determine your position by the best means available, and include this position in your radio messages. If position is based on celestial observations, transmit the observations also.
- If you have bailed out, try to make your way to the crashed plane. Rescuers can spot it from the air even when they cannot see a man.
- Stay with the airplane unless briefed to the contrary. Do not leave the airplane unless you know that you are within easy walking distance of help. If you travel, leave a note giving planned

route. Stick to your plan so rescuers can locate you.

You are the key man in the rescue. Help the search parties to find you, and follow their instructions when they sight you. They can use all the assistance you can give. Don't take chances which might result in injury. You will be easier to rescue if you are in one piece.

The following procedures will speed up your rescue:

- *Conserve power of electronic equipment. Use it according to procedures given in your briefing.*
- *Sweep the horizon with your signal mirror at frequent intervals.*

First Aid

GENERAL

The most likely injuries will be cuts and bruises, fractures, brain concussion, internal injuries, and burns. Keep injured men lying down. Place unconscious men face down with head turned to one side. Those with head injuries should lie flat on their backs with head level or raised. Handle patients very carefully. Watch for symptoms of shock. Keep patients warm.

When there is no chance that an injured person can be treated by medical personnel within a short period, the treatment rendered must be final treatment. *The primary aim is to prevent loss of life and either to prepare the injured party for movement or to be less of a problem to his companions or to himself.*

You must be prepared to treat your own injuries. These injuries may be simple or, in some cases, so severe that death could result unless you act to preclude it. Simple, temporary treatment of injuries under these circumstances would be to no avail. You must be prepared to undertake strong measures to sustain life.

BLEEDING. Place sterile pad directly on wound and apply pressure by hand or by bandaging firmly.

Elevate an arm or leg if bleeding does not stop, provided you think no bones are broken.

Use a tourniquet only if a limb is badly crushed, blood is gushing from a wound, or if bleeding is not stopped by a pressure bandage. Place the tourniquet on upper arm or leg between injury and heart. Leave the tourniquet in place until the bleeder has been tied off; if bleeder cannot be tied off, leave the tourniquet in place until physiological amputation is complete. Keep the treatment area as warm as possible.

CONTROL OF BLEEDING. Serious bleeding must be controlled at once. In only a few minutes, life can ebb away; and without the ability to replace the blood, the life is lost.

Direct pressure compresses will stop most bleeding. Use of a tourniquet under such circumstances may sacrifice a limb or, if improperly applied, may increase the bleeding. Application of strong pressure may be required until the seriously bleeding vessel can be tied off with thread or a fine string. If reasonably sure that the bleeder is in a given bit of tissue, the entire area can be tied off, thus stopping the bleeder. This may be done by using a large needle to pass into the tissue and around the area of severe bleeding and tying the entire mass securely.

CESSATION OF BREATHING. The best form of artificial respiration is the mouth-to-mouth type. It is the only technique which guarantees enough air exchange to revive the unconscious person, and allows the "operator" to insure that the airway is open. If there is an obstruction, air cannot enter the lungs regardless of the method of artificial respiration used.

There are three main causes for obstruction:

1. Liquid, false teeth, or other foreign matter in the mouth or throat.
2. Relaxation of the jaw. The tongue is attached to the jaw so that it falls backward and blocks the throat (called "swallowing the tongue").
3. Position of the neck. When the neck is bent forward so that the chin is near the chest, the throat becomes "kinked" and blocks the passage of air.

To correct any of the above conditions, place the patient on his back looking upwards and hold the lower jaw forward.

Procedure

1. Turn the victim on his back.
2. Clean the mouth, nose, and throat. If the mouth, nose, and throat appear clean, start exhaled-air artificial respiration immediately. If foreign matter such as vomitus or mucus is visible in the mouth, nose, and throat, wipe it away quickly with a cloth or by passing the index and middle fingers through the throat in a sweeping motion.
3. Place the victim's head in the "sword-swallowing" position. The head must be placed as far back as possible so that the front of the neck is stretched.
4. Hold the lower jaw up. Approach the victim's head, preferably from his left side. Insert the thumb of your left hand between the victim's teeth at the midline. Pull the lower jaw forcefully outward so that the lower teeth are further forward than the upper teeth. Hold the jaw in this position as long as the victim is unconscious. A piece of cloth may be wrapped around your thumb to prevent injury by the victim's teeth.
5. Close the nose. Close the victim's nose by compressing it between the thumb and forefinger of the right hand.
6. Blow air into the victim's open mouth with your open mouth with airtight contact. Blow rapidly and forcefully until the chest rises.
7. Let air out of victim's lungs. After chest rises, quickly separate lip contact with the victim, and allow the victim to exhale by himself.

If the chest did not rise when you blew in, improve the support of the victim's air passageway, and blow more forcefully. Repeat the inflations of the lungs 12 to 20 times per minute. You'll need to breathe slightly deeper and faster than usual to get enough air for yourself, but don't worry about this point. Continue rhythmically without interruption until the victim starts breathing or is obviously dead. A smooth rhythm is desirable, but split-second timing is not essential.

If the victim appears to be breathing to some degree, keep his air passageway open until he awakens by maintaining the support of his lower jaw. If his tongue or fingernails are blue rather than pink, he is not breathing adequately and requires assistance.

Although the victim may appear to be breathing because of movement of his chest and abdomen, air may not be moving into his lungs due to complete obstruction of the air passageway from improper positioning of the head and jaw. For this reason, it is most important to determine whether or not there is any movement of air in and out of the mouth and nose by listening closely.

HEART STOPPAGE. If the heart has stopped, external cardiac massage (manual heart compression) must be given simultaneously with mouth-to-mouth resuscitation.

1. A few puffs of air should immediately be given by mouth-to-mouth resuscitation as above. (It should be continued by another person; but if there is no one else, you can interrupt massage every 15 to 30 seconds to fill the lungs with air two or three times and then return to the massage.)
2. Place yourself on your patient's right with your left hand on the lower third of his sternum (breastbone) so that the heel of that hand will deliver the pressure. Rest your right hand on the left, fingers pointing to his chin. Your position should be such that your body weight can be used in applying pressure.
3. Apply pressure vertically, downward, approximately once per second so that the patient's sternum moves one and a half to two inches toward his spine.
4. At the end of each stroke, lift your hands so that his chest will expand fully by recoil.
5. After heart action has resumed, manual heart compression should be continued until pulse is strong.

CHEST WOUNDS. Open chest wounds, through which air can be heard sucking, should be covered with a large dressing. Air entering the wound allows the lungs to collapse. Expansion of rib cage and movement of diaphragm (muscle wall between chest cavity and abdomen) causes air to enter through the wound instead of through normal air passages. Consequently, the pad should be firmly applied at the moment of maximum exhalation, just before more air is sucked in. It should be firm enough to make a seal, but not tight enough to stop chest movement entirely.

SHOCK. All personnel are likely to suffer some shock after an emergency landing. Men in shock may have pale, cold skin; they may sweat, breathe rapidly, and have a weak pulse; they may be confused or unconscious.

Lay the patient down flat, with feet raised.

Keep him warm, but not overheated. If he is conscious and not injured internally, give him warm drinks; *do not give alcohol.*

Give oxygen if it is available.

If the patient is in severe pain from injury, give a morphine injection (syrette) according to directions on the container. (Always give the injection above the tourniquet, or on the uninjured extremity.) Do not give morphine to a person who is unconscious, in deep shock, wounded in the chest and having breathing difficulties, or who is suffering from a broken neck or severe head injuries. Remember, *use morphine with caution.*

Be reassuring and cheerful with men in shock.

EYE INJURY. Clean wound and eye by irrigating with clean water. Apply ophthalmic (eye) ointment or antibiotic ointment such as penicillin, terramycin, etc., when available. Cover eye with clean dressing. Give aspirin for pain.

To remove a foreign body from the eye, first irrigate with clean water. If not successful, then wind sterile cotton on a match stick to make an applicator. Moisten with clean water and attempt to dislodge the foreign body by several gentle swipes over the affected area. If this is unsuccessful, make no further attempt to remove it; just apply ointment.

FRACTURES AND DISLOCATIONS. Handle injured men with care to avoid causing them more injury.

Don't remove clothing from a fractured limb. If a wound exists, cut away clothing and treat before splinting. Clothing is most easily cut at the seams.

Give a morphine injection (syrette) for severe pain (except for head injuries and other cases in which morphine may not be used).

Keep the patient lying quiet; don't move him.

The treatment of fractures is normally considered beyond the scope of first aid; however, in the prolonged survival situation, the correction of bone deformities is necessary to hasten healing and to obtain the result that will allow the injured party to use the injured member. The best time for manipulating a fracture is immediately following the injury, before painful muscle spasm sets in. Traction should be applied until overriding fragments of bone are brought into line (check by comparing with other limb). Then firmly immobilize the extremity.

An immobilization device must be constructed. This may be done by weaving together willow branches or other stable items to form a splint-cast. Temporary splints may be improvised from pieces of equipment or from a tight roll of clothing; pad with soft materials. The splint should be long enough to incorporate the joints above and below the fracture.

Gentle but firm traction is also applied to extremities to reduce dislocations.

If you are alone, the problem of treating fractures or dislocations is more complicated but not impossible, for traction can be applied by using gravity. The wrist or ankle end of the extremity can be tied to (or wedged into) a fork of a tree or similar point of firm fixation. The weight of the body is then allowed to exert the necessary counter-traction with the joint being manipulated until the dislocation (or fracture) is treated. Before beginning the procedure, necessary splinting materials must be collected and be readily available.

SPRAINS. Bandage and keep sprained part at rest. Application of local cold may prevent swelling. When swelling has decreased (in 6 to 8 hours), application of local heat will ease pain. Elevate the injured extremity.

If it is necessary to use the sprained limb, immobilize the injured area as much as possible with a splint or heavy wrapping. If no broken bones are involved, a sprained limb can be used.

TO PREVENT INFECTION. Cut away clothing necessary to get at a wound. Don't touch a wound with fingers or dirty objects. Don't suck wounds, except snake bites, and then only if there are no cuts or sores in your mouth.

Apply sterile dressing with firm pressure into wound. Tie firmly but not too tightly.

Keep wounded part at rest.

Iodine may be used to sterilize skin areas surrounding a wound but should not be poured directly into an open wound. Let iodine dry in air before applying bandage.

BURNS. One of the most frequent survival or aircraft emergency injuries is burns. Burns cause severe pain, often result in shock and infection, and offer an avenue for the loss of body fluid and salts. The initial treatment is directed toward the relief of pain and prevention of infection. In survival, the closed method of treatment has certain advantages. Covering the wound with a clean dressing of any type reduces the pain and the chances of infection. Further, such protection enhances mobility and performance of vital survival functions.

Maintenance of body fluids and salts is essential to the recovery from burns. Administer fluids by mouth. Drink quantities of water following the burn damage. If possible, add salt (2 tablets per canteenful) to the water. Three or more canteens or water should be drunk every 24 hours.

Don't touch a burned part with fingers. Apply thick gauze pack; bandage firmly. Don't change bandage. If pain is severe, give a morphine injection. Keep the burned part at rest. Splints may sometimes be used to good advantage.

ARCTIC

Keep injured men warm and dry. Put the patient in sleeping bag, provide shelter, and build a fire. Warm food and liquids are desirable for conscious patients. Avoid alcohol. Improvise heat packs by heating rocks, sand, metal, or dirt, and wrapping it in fabric. Place packs at the small of the back, between thighs, under armpits, on stomach, and on soles of feet, or as the patient requests. *Make sure not to burn the skin.*

FROSTBITE. Frostbite is the freezing of some part of the body. It is a constant hazard in sub-zero operations, especially when the wind is strong. As a rule, the first sensation of frostbite is numbness rather than pain. You can see the effects of frostbite, a grayish or yellow-white spot on the skin, before you can feel it.

Use the buddy system. Watch your buddy's face to see if any frozen spots show; and have him watch yours.

Get the frostbite casualty into a heated shelter if possible.

When only the surface skin is frozen (frost nip or superficial frostbite), it becomes "spongy" to the touch. It can be rewarmed by body heat. If deeper tissues are involved (deep frozen), the thawing process must take place quickly. Ideally, thawing is accomplished in warm water. Because refreezing of a thawed part means certain loss of tissue, it is better, in some cases, to continue with a frozen part as it is rather than to thaw it when there is a chance of refreezing. Thawing must, however, be accomplished as soon as possible.

Warm the frozen part rapidly. Frozen parts should be thawed in water until soft, even though the treatment is painful. This treatment is most effective when the water is between 105°F and 110°F (comfortably warm to a normally protected part such as an elbow). If warm water is not available, wrap the frozen part in blankets or clothing and apply improvised heat packs. Thawed extremities should be immobilized.

Use body heat to aid in thawing. Hold a bare, warm palm against frostbitten ears or parts of the face. Grasp a frostbitten wrist with a warm, bare hand. Hold frostbitten hands against the chest, under the armpits, or between the legs at the groin. Hold a frostbitten foot against a companion's stomach or between his thighs.

When frostbite is accompanied by breaks in the skin, apply sterile dressing. Do not use strong antiseptics such as tincture of iodine. Do not use powdered sulfa drugs in the wound.

Never forcibly remove frozen shoes and mittens. Place in lukewarm water until soft and then remove gently.

Never rub frostbite. You may tear frozen tissues and cause further tissue damage. Never apply snow or ice; that just increases the cold injury. Never soak frozen limbs in kerosene or oil.

Do not try to thaw a frozen part by exercising. Exercise of frozen parts will increase tissue damage and is likely to break the skin. Do not stand or walk on frozen feet. You will only cause tissue damage.

IMMERSION FOOT (TRENCH FOOT). Immersion foot is a cold injury resulting from prolonged exposure to temperatures just above freezing. In the early stages of immersion foot, your feet and toes are pale and feel cold, numb, and stiff. Walking becomes difficult. If you do not take preventive action at this state, your feet will swell and become very painful. In extreme cases of immersion foot, your flesh dies, and amputation of the foot or of the leg may be necessary.

Because the early stages are not very painful, you must be constantly alert to prevent the development of immersion foot. To prevent this condition:

Keep your feet dry by wearing waterproof footgear and keeping your shelter dry.

Clean and dry your socks and shoes at every opportunity.

Dry your feet as soon as possible after getting them wet.

Warm them with your hands, apply foot powder, and put on dry socks.

When you must wear wet socks and shoes, exercise your feet continually by wriggling your toes and bending your ankles. If you sleep in a sitting position, put on dry socks, warm your feet, and elevate your legs as high as possible. Do not wear tight shoes.

Treat immersion foot by keeping the affected part dry and warm. If possible, keep the foot and leg in a horizontal position to increase circulation.

SEVERE CHILLING. If you are totally immersed in cold water for even a few minutes, your body temperature will drop. Long exposures to severe dry cold on land can also lower your body temperature. The only remedy for this severe chilling is warming of the entire body. Warm by any means available. The preferred treatment is warming in a hot bath. Severe chilling may be accompanied by shock.

SNOWBLINDNESS. Symptoms of snowblindness are redness, burning, watering, or sandy-feeling eyes, the halo one sees when looking at lights, headaches, and poor vision. Remember that snowblindness may not appear until 4–6 hours after exposure. For this reason, it is often not suspected because the symptoms do not appear until well after sunset.

Treat snowblindness by protecting the eyes from light and relieving the pain. Protect the eyes by staying in a dark shelter or by wearing a lightproof bandage. Relieve the pain by putting cold compresses on the eyes, if there is no danger of freezing, and by taking aspirin. Use no eye drops or ointment. Most cases recover within 18 hours without medical treatment. The first attack of snowblindness makes the victim susceptible to future attacks.

CARBON MONOXIDE POISONING. Carbon monoxide poisoning can be caused by a fire burning in an unventilated shelter. Usually there are no symptoms; unconsciousness and death may occur without previous warning. Sometimes, however, there may be pressure at the temples, headache, pounding pulse, drowsiness, and nausea. Treat by getting into fresh air at once; keep warm and at rest. If necessary, apply artificial respiration. Give oxygen if available.

DESERT

Exposure to the desert sun can be dangerous. It can cause three types of heat collapse.

HEAT CRAMPS. The first warning of heat collapse usually is cramps in leg or belly muscles. Keep the patient resting; give him salt dissolved in water.

HEAT EXHAUSTION. Patient is first flushed, then pale, sweats heavily, has moist, cool skin, and may become delirious or unconscious.

Treat the patient by placing him in the shade, flat on his back. Give him salt dissolved in water—two tablets to a canteen.

HEAT STROKE. Heat stroke may come on suddenly. The face is red, skin hot and dry. All sweating stops. There is severe headache; pulse is fast and strong. Unconsciousness may result.

Treat the patient by cooling him off. Loosen his clothing; lay him down flat, but off the ground, in the shade. Cool by saturating his clothes with water and by fanning. Do not give stimulants.

TROPICS

WOUNDS. Even the smallest scratch can quickly become dangerously infected in the tropics. Promptly disinfect any wound.

SNAKEBITE. If you are bitten, immediately apply a constriction band (tourniquet) only tight enough to shut off venous, i.e., return, flow of the blood between the snakebite and the heart. Then make a single cut parallel to the long axis of the limb about one-quarter inch deep through each fang mark and immediately apply suction over the bite—by mouth if there are no open sores in the mouth, and spit out poison immediately. In the moist tropics, instead of making the cuts, use deep massage with the teeth combined with strong oral suction. Immobilize and splint the injured member. Apply cool compresses to reduce pain, and remain quiet as much as possible. *Don't give alcohol!*

If you lose your shoes or they wear out, you can improvise a practical pair of sandals by using the rubber sidewall of a tire or a piece of bark for the soles, with a parachute cloth or canvas for the uppers and heel straps.

Dry your clothing before nightfall to avoid discomfort from cold.

If you have an extra change of clothes, especially socks, keep it dry to replace wet clothing.

Wash clothing, especially socks, daily. Dirty clothes not only rot but may lead to skin diseases.

Clothes which have been removed should be hung up. If laid on the ground, they may collect ants, scorpions, or snakes. Always check footgear and clothing for such "guests" before putting it on.

Health and Hazards

GENERAL

Keeping well is especially important when you are stranded on your own. Your physical condition will have a lot to do with your coming out safely. Protection against heat and cold and knowledge of how to find water and food are important to your health. But there are more rules you should follow:

Drink enough water to avoid dehydration. If water is scarce or difficult to obtain, avoid excessive dehydration from sweating.

Save your strength. Avoid fatigue. Get enough sleep. Even if you can't sleep at first, lie down, relax, loosen up. Stop worrying; learn to take it easy. If you are doing hard work or walking, rest for 10 minutes each hour.

Take care of your feet. Your feet are important, especially if you are going to walk. If your feet hurt, stop and take care of them; it will save you trouble later on. Examine your feet when you first stop to see if there are any red spots or blisters.

Apply adhesive tape smoothly on your skin where shoes rub. If you have a blister, it is best to leave it intact. This will decrease chances of infection. If it is broken or punctured, don't remove the protective skin over the blister. Apply a sterile dressing.

Guard against skin infection. Your skin is the first line of defense against infection. Use an antiseptic on even the smallest scratch, cut, or insect bite. Keep your fingernails cut short to prevent infection from scratching. Cuts and scratches are apt to get seriously infected, especially in the tropics. A bad infection may hurt your chance of coming out safely.

Guard against intestinal sickness. Diarrhea and other intestinal sickness may be caused by change of water and food, contaminated water or spoiled food, excess fatigue, overeating in hot weather, or using dirty dishes. Purify all water used for drinking, either by purification tablets or by boiling for one minute plus an additional minute for every thousand feet of altitude. Cook the plants you eat, or wash them carefully with purified water. Make a habit of personal cleanliness; wash your hands with soap and water, if possible, before eating. If one member of your group gets diarrhea, take special care to enforce measures for proper disposal of human waste and to insure cleanliness in handling food and water. Field treatment of diarrhea is necessarily limited. Rest and fast—except for drinking water—for 24 hours; then take only liquid foods such as soup and tea, and avoid sugars and starches. Keep up a large intake of water, with salt tablets. Eat several meals instead of one or two large ones.

Don't worry about lack of bowel movement, this will take care of itself in a few days if you exercise and drink plenty of water.

Keep your body and clothing clean. You will feel better and keep free from skin infections and body parasites. Examine each other for external parasites.

Keep your camp clean. Dump garbage in a pit or in a spot away from camp where it will not blow about. Dig a latrine or designate a latrine area away from the camp water supply.

Water

GENERAL

Water is one of your first and most important needs. Start looking for it immediately. You can get along for weeks without food, but *you can't live long without water*, especially in hot areas.

Even in cold areas, your body needs 2 quarts of water a day to maintain efficiency. Any lower intake results in loss of efficiency. If you delay drinking, you will have to make it up later on. Dehydration can be just as serious a problem in cold areas as in the desert. Don't neglect it.

Purify all water before drinking, either (1) by boiling for at least one minute plus an additional minute for each thousand feet of altitude; or (2) by using the water purification tablets in your first aid or survival kit according to instructions; or (3) by adding 8 drops of 2½% tincture of iodine to a quart (canteenful) of water and letting it stand for 10 minutes before drinking. Rainwater collected directly in clean containers or in plants is generally safe to drink without purifying.

Don't drink urine or sea water—the salt content is too high.

GROUND WATER. When no surface water is available, you may want to tap the underground water supply. Access to this water supply depends upon the kind of ground—whether it is rocky or of some loose material like clay, gravel, or sand.

ROCK. In rocky ground look for springs and seepages. Limestones and lavas have more and larger springs than any other rocks. Springs of cold water are safest; warm water has been recently at the surface and is more likely to be polluted.

Limestones are soluble; and ground water etches out waterways and caverns in them. Look in these caverns, large and small, for springs. If you go into a large one beyond sight of the entrance, be careful—don't get lost.

Most lava rocks contain millions of bubble-holes; ground water may seep through them. Look for springs along the walls of valleys that cross the lava flow. Some flows have no bubbles but do have "organ pipe" joints—vertical cracks that part the rocks into columns a foot or more thick and 20 feet or more high. At the foot of these joints, you may find water creeping out as seepage or pouring out in springs.

Look for seepage where a dry canyon cuts through a layer of porous sandstone.

Index